Diamonds And Stones In An Era Of Gold

Brian Collopy AM

16

EasyRead Large

RHYW

Copyright Page from the Original Book

Glass House Books
an imprint of IP (Interactive Publications Pty Ltd)
Treetop Studio • 9 Kuhler Court
Carindale, Queensland, Australia 4152
sales@ipoz.biz
ipoz.biz/ipstore

First published by IP in 2018

Printed in 12 pt Book Antiqua on 14 pt Bookman Old Style.

National Library of Australia
Cataloguing-in-Publication entry:

Creator:	Brian Collopy AM – author
Title:	Diamonds and stones in an era of gold / Brian Collopy AM.
ISBN:	9781925231656 (paperback) 9781925231663 (eBook)
Notes:	Includes bibliographical references
Subjects:	Medical History Melbourne, History Legal History Dr James Beaney

TABLE OF CONTENTS

Diamonds and Stones in an Era of Gold

Brian T. Collopy graduated M.B.B.S. Melbourne and holds Fellowships of the Royal Australasian College of Surgeons, the Royal College of Surgeons of England and the Royal Australasian College of Medical Administrators. He is a past Director of the Department of Colon and Rectal Surgery at St. Vincent's Hospital, Melbourne and Associate Professor of Surgery at Melbourne University. He has had a long-standing interest in the assessment of the quality of care and with the award of a Kellogg Fellowship, and subsequently a WHO consultancy, he studied and advised on health care practices in Europe and Asia, as well as North America.

He has conducted numerous studies addressing the quality of care at the hospital, inter-hospital and national levels, has authored or co-authored over 150 papers published in peer-reviewed journals, and has spoken extensively on the subject.

Amongst a variety of roles in relation to the quality of health care he was President of the Australian Council on Healthcare Standards (ACHS), which conducts a national hospital accreditation program. With ACHS he developed clinical performance measures, which are now used in a number of other countries, and provide the ACHS with a unique national clinical database. Other offices include being Chairman of the Advisory Council of the International Society of

Quality Assurance (ISQua) and the Advisory Committee on Elective Surgery (ACES) in Victoria.

He was made a Member of the Order of Australia in 1993 and received a Fellowship of the Australian Medical Association in 1996.

Currently he is the Director of CQM Consultants, formed to assist health care organisations to assess the quality of their care. In this capacity he has guided tertiary referral hospitals on performance measurement and assisted organisations such as the Department of Health in South Australia, the Royal Flying Doctor Service, Correctional Health Services, and New South Wales Mental Health. He has also assisted the Hong Kong Hospital Authority to develop clinical performance measures.

He has just retired from membership of the Victorian Civil & Administrative Tribunal (VCAT), but continues as a Clinical Advisor to the ACHS and as a member of the Superannuation Complaints Tribunal (SCT).

A number of his activities, such as the clinical indicator development for hospital accreditation, a follow-up protocol after bowel cancer surgery, and the categorisation of urgency for elective surgery waiting list patients, were world-first achievements.

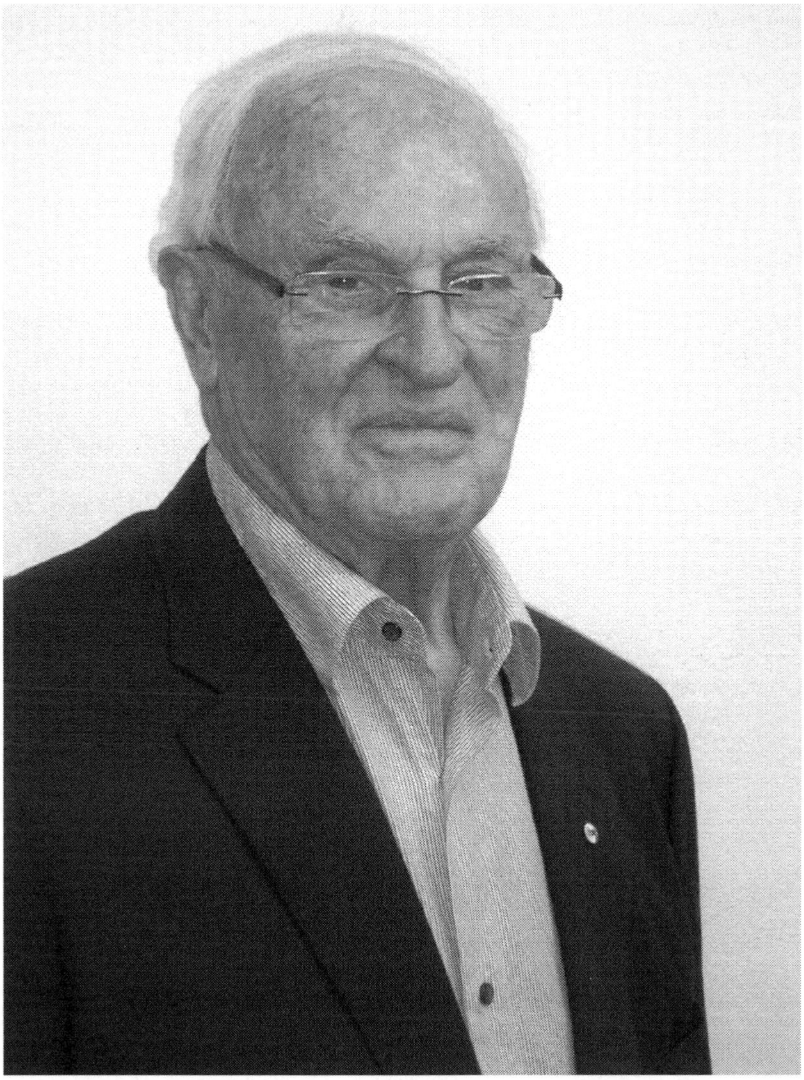

Acknowledgements

Cover image: Cate Collopy

The image of James L. Purves (p.96) is with the permission of the Victorian Bar and appeared in the *Victorian Bar News* 113.

Other images are from the author's private collection, and, despite his best efforts, their original sources cannot be identified.

Foreword

The title of this book reflects both life at the time in Melbourne and the main figure of the book, namely James Beaney. Brian Collopy, the author, has been a close colleague and friend of mine for many years. More importantly he has been a distinguished Melbourne surgeon, very involved in the measurement of surgical outcomes and the assessment of patient safety. Who then could be better qualified to evaluate the life of James Beaney, over 100 years after his time?

James Beaney was a flamboyant character both in surgery and in Melbourne's social life. He was known as "Diamond Jim" or "Champagne Jimmy" as he wore many diamond rings (not removed when operating). Champagne, which he dispensed liberally, was the favourite tipple for him at any time but also for his team after surgery.

He was born in Kent in 1828 of working class parents. He was educated in Canterbury and after apprenticeship to a chemist, and then a surgeon, he enrolled for medical studies at Edinburgh. However, he developed tuberculosis, which was not responding to rest, so he set off to Melbourne in 1852 to further his progress to health. In Melbourne, he worked for a chemist in Collins Street and then returned to England to pursue his medical studies at Edinburgh. He became MRCS and later, in 1860, was awarded an FRCS of the Edinburgh College of Surgery. He then returned to Melbourne where he was a locum in the very lucrative practice of Dr. John Maund, which subsequently he inherited.

He was elected to the Melbourne Hospital as an Honorary Consultant Surgeon for the first time around 1860 and for a second time in 1875. The election to the consultant staff at the Melbourne was dictated by the number of votes given by patients and supporters of the hospital and it is said that he spent considerable money in advertising, and no doubt dispensed much champagne on achieving his consultant status.

The portrayal of Melbourne in the second part of the 19th century is fascinating. It had been described by a visiting journalist from the UK as 'Marvellous Melbourne', and was probably one of the most affluent cities in the world at that time, as a result of the Bendigo and Ballarat gold rushes.

As a surgeon, Beaney was a bold advocate of his discipline, particularly in paediatric surgery and sexually transmitted disease. But he was very much a self-promoter and so many of the medical profession in Melbourne were adamantly opposed to Beaney. He had a very large private practice and was probably the wealthiest surgeon in the colonies. The home that he built on the corner of Collins and Russell Streets (pictured in the book) was a four-storey mansion, which included his consulting rooms, his residence, an operating room and a roof garden!

He was involved in several major legal trials; the first one described by Collopy was of a young barmaid who died of a ruptured uterus, which was allegedly due to an abortion. He was acquitted after a re-trial, the jury having been split at the first one. A subsequent major trial, which Collopy records in detail, concerns the death of a patient following removal of a very large bladder stone with a charge of negligence on Beaney's part. His defence was conducted by a young barrister, James Purves. The efforts of Purves were quite remarkable and this makes entertaining reading for, perhaps amazingly, Purves had Beaney acquitted of manslaughter.

Beaney was also was a great philanthropist. One major legacy was to Canterbury in that he left money to establish the "Beaney Institute for the Education of the Working Man", reflecting perhaps his own origins. This today is a flourishing library and museum of the history of Canterbury and is known in Canterbury as The Beaney. He also left several bequests to the University of Melbourne and the Medical School, and the Beaney Prize in Surgery continues to this day. It must be said that neither the author nor the person writing this Foreword won the Beaney Prize!

Overall, this is one of the most interesting and enjoyable books I have read for some time and it will appeal to all. Beaney was a colourful character in a booming time in Melbourne and this has been brought splendidly to life by Brian Collopy in *Diamonds and Stones in an Era of Gold.*

– Professor Sir Peter Morris, AC, FRS, FRCS

Nuffield Professor of Surgery Emeritus, University of Oxford Fellow Emeritus of Balliol College, University of Oxford Past President of the Royal College of Surgeons of England

Introduction

In the Melbourne General Cemetery in Carlton a monument to the surgeon Dr James Beaney, who died on 30 June 1891, towers over those surrounding it. There is also a set of memorial tablets to him in England in the Canterbury Cathedral and an historical museum in the city of Canterbury known locally as the 'Beaney'. For the former he had left a sum of £1000 for the restoration of the cathedral, and the museum was originally developed from £10,000 he provided in his will for the establishment of 'The Beaney Institute for the Education of the Working Man'. At Melbourne University there was a Beaney Prize in Surgery, which for many years was awarded annually to the final year medical student who was outstanding in the surgical examination. It is now awarded as a scholarship to a graduate engaged in surgical research at one of the three clinical schools attached to Melbourne University. There is a similar scholarship in pathology. He was the first benefactor to the University of Melbourne Medical School, which had been founded in 1862.

Few people who have viewed the monument would have known what a colourful and controversial surgeon Dr. James Beaney was in his dress and adornments, in his surgical beliefs and writing and in the considerable litigious events in which he was the central player. Certainly none of my surgical colleagues or teachers could match him for those characteristics, nor it appears could any of his contemporaries in Melbourne in the second half of the 19th century.

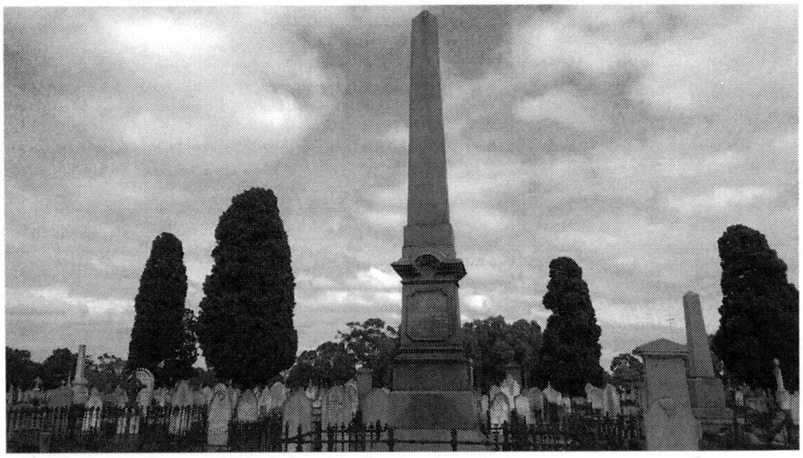

Figure 1: Monument to Dr. James Beaney, Melbourne General Cemetery, Carlton.

In addition to many years spent in surgical practice in a University teaching hospital and in a major private hospital I have been involved, at a local, national and international level, in the assessment of the standards of patient care and in the development of formal measures to enable such assessments. Many of my activities in this area have been published in peer-reviewed health care journals, but this is the first time I have written about an individual medical practitioner.

It was while researching the history of hospital infection rates (for comparison with current data) that I came across a newspaper article from 1886 strongly criticising the report of a Victorian Parliamentary committee, which had found no fault with the infection rates or with patient management practices at the Melbourne Hospital. The chairman of the committee was James Beaney, and the accusatory article made it quite clear that he was protecting his own interests. That encouraged me to learn more about him.

Seeing Beaney's name reminded me also that some years beforehand a colleague had given me a small book he had found in his late father's possessions. It was a monograph, published in Melbourne in 1876 by an F.F. Bailliere, and had a long title: *Lithotomy: Its successes and dangers. Being a verbatim report, from shorthand notes, of an inquest, held before the City Coroner with a preface and commentary by an MRCSE.* Its author, listed as MRCSE, is believed to be this extraordinary surgeon James George Beaney himself. It was said to have cost £700 to produce, a significant sum at that time. The book was never sold but copies were distributed throughout Melbourne. The monograph, as its title implies, is a report of an inquest, held late in 1875, into the death of a patient upon whom James Beaney had operated. It provided an account of the conduct of the inquest and the brilliant defence of Beaney by a young barrister named James Purves. An assessment of James Purves in Sir Arthur Dean's book *A Multitude of Counsellors – A History of the Victorian Bar* (1968), in which he described Purves as 'Undoubtedly the greatest advocate the Victorian Bar has produced', increased my interest to learn more about the particular episode, the players involved and the circumstances, both social and professional, of that period in Melbourne.

The accuracy of the account of this particular inquest is verified by reports in the newspapers of that time, particularly those in the *Argus* and *The Age,* in which the details of the inquest corresponded closely with those in the monograph, and also by a review of the limited 'proceedings' available from the Public Records Office.

I have considerably expanded on the court dialogue in the 1875 inquest and provided information on the various players in a drama, which was lacking in the monograph. I have provided reasons why the inquest was held, a principal one being an indiscreet shop window display of a surgical specimen, organised by Beaney. Without this display an incensed and unknown surgeon, who claimed further knowledge of the operating circumstances in the particular case that was the concern of the inquest, might not have been provoked to make a public response.

I have also described the equally extraordinary place that Melbourne was then. While lacking the modern forms of communication, information sharing and transport, the pace of change in Melbourne was frenetic, as this 'faraway' city grew into one of the grandest in the English-speaking world of that time. The growth was due, of course, to the immense amount of gold extracted from the mid-Victorian fields at Ballarat and Bendigo, not far to the north of

Melbourne. This should help the reader understand how the idiosyncratic James Beaney could be accepted (or tolerated by some) in the city at that time, obtain a senior surgical position in the Melbourne Hospital and develop such a large private surgical practice.

An aggressive attitude existed between many medical practitioners of that period in Melbourne. This had something to do with the fact that, prior to 1867, all doctors in the Colonies had qualified overseas (usually England, Scotland or Ireland). Many were adventurers who came out to seek their fortune at the gold diggings or elsewhere. Not finding their pots of gold, they reverted to medical practice.

Back then, they often found they were competing against charlatans, with bogus degrees, who used bizarre, and frequently dangerous, treatments on patients who had little medical knowledge. The *Medical Act of 1865* in England had had a minimal effect in reducing false claims of cure and the advertising of non-existent medical skills. Criticism of the 'healing profession' was rife, and it was common, even for legitimate practitioners, to have their credentials questioned. They had to be alert and wary and, as a result, were often defensive and frequently aggressive.

A further stress factor was the enormous amount of litigation surrounding surgery in that period of limited knowledge and an absence of modern diagnostic and support services. An example was the case in 1871 of a woman who suffered injuries to her knee and hip. A Dr. Van Hemert, a well-known and respected Melbourne practitioner, missed a fracture of the neck of her femur (thigh bone) and was sued. In the resulting court case James Beaney gave evidence for the plaintiff, who won her case. At a subsequent special meeting of the Medical Society of Victoria, a motion was passed declaring the decision unfair and wrong. Dr. Beaney arrived at that meeting late and was not permitted to explain the reasons for his damming evidence. He had apparently resigned from the Society the year before. The Medical Society's motion could not, of course, reverse the court decision. Dr. Van Hemert was reported to be 'broken in spirit' and left the country. He would have avoided the mishap if x-rays had been available, but Professor Wilhelm Roentgen of Bavaria did not make his remarkable radiological discovery until 1895.

The advent of anaesthetic agents in the 1840s had led to a rapid increase in the number and complexity of surgical procedures by that time, as with the patient 'asleep' and not screaming, the need for surgical speed was reduced. An example of the speed required in the absence of general anaesthesia was evident in a report of an amputation of a leg, above the knee, performed in the Hobart Hospital in the 1840s. The time from the first incision to removal of the limb was just three minutes.

With anaesthesia, various operations upon body cavities and organs could then be performed. However, these new procedures, as well as the more traditional operations, were associated with high complication rates and consequently also high mortality rates. The antibacterial drug era was still many decades away and as post-operative infection was an enormous problem reference to sepsis is included in this narrative.

The relatively small number of surgeons in Melbourne then were frequently called upon to give evidence for or against their colleagues and the proceedings were generally made public by an unsympathetic press, which took delight in disclosing the shortcomings of those who "wielded the knife". The pen and the tongue were powerful weapons. A loose comment from one's colleague, when picked up by a journalist, could cut short a promising medical practice, providing another reason for resentment and mistrust to abound in the colony's healing profession.

The first word, lithotomy, in the monograph's title, refers to the operation for removal of a bladder stone or stones by cutting into the bladder. Hippocrates, over 2000 years ago, had recognised the risks to life associated with lithotomy, and part of his oath included: 'I will not cut for stone, even for the patients in whom the disease is manifest; I will leave this operation to be performed by practitioners.' This was probably the first mention of specialist surgeons, the appropriate specialist branch of surgery today being known as urology.

Mention of operations for bladder stone can be found in Arabian, Greek and Roman history. Early descriptions also indicate that there could be a 'low' and a 'high' approach to the stone, the former being lithotomy via the perineum (as was the approach in the case relevant to the monograph) and the latter being suprapubic (lower abdominal). The low or perineal lithotomy, as will unfold for the reader, could be performed by a median approach, i.e. a surgical incision made in the midline, or by a lateral approach. It was doubtful whether there was any clear advantage to avoiding the midline. The significant understanding quickly reached by the barrister defending Dr. Beaney about the intricacies of lithotomy and its consequences will be evident to the readers.

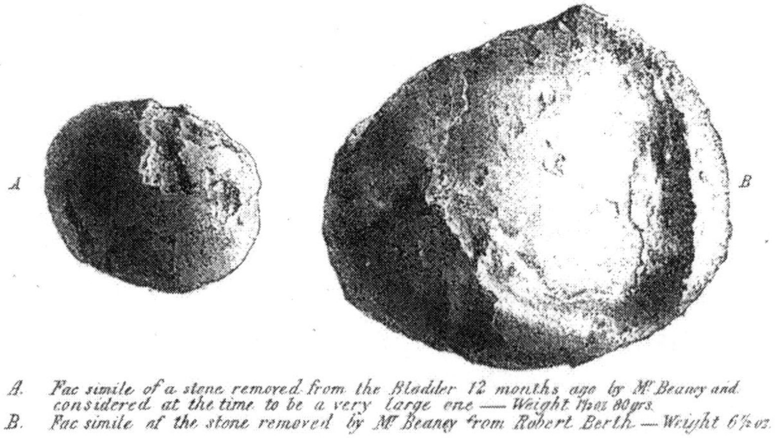

Figure 2: Facsimile of the Bladder Stone removed by Dr. Beaney.

1. Re-election

Character is like a tree and a reputation like its shadow. The shadow is what we think of it, the tree is the real thing. – Abraham Lincoln

The surgeon James Beaney's re-election to the Melbourne Hospital in 1875, a decade after he had been dropped from the list of attending surgeons, was met with disapproval by several of his colleagues and by others involved in the hospital's affairs. There were a number of reasons for this. Many were annoyed that he should claim that he was now the "senior"surgeon because he had topped the surgical voting, for there was no such position, and there was disappointment that he had displaced a good staff member. There was also concern that, because of past events surrounding Beaney, the reputation of the hospital might be jeopardised, but more about that shortly.

The principal reason for resentment, bordering on hostility, related to Beaney's pre-election behaviour. Beaney had campaigned hard for re-election to the hospital staff. His textbook publisher, F.F. Baillière, had distributed coloured leaflets to the Melbourne Hospital's subscribers three weeks before they were due to vote on the staff elections. The leaflets had outlined Beaney's publications, including what he claimed to be the first surgical textbook in Australia.

Its title was *Original Contributions to the Practice of Conservative Surgery.* Baillière, with his knowledge of Beaney's reputation, had intentionally included "conservative" in the title as it suggested a careful and caring surgeon. Ballière and Beaney worked well together although, in later years, they were to have a falling out, shortly before the former's tragic death in a Jolimont railway accident.

Whilst this unacceptable advertising might not upset more secure surgical colleagues such as Thomas Fitzgerald, it served to irritate Edward Barker, who had replaced Beaney on the honorary surgical staff in 1865. Ten years later, Beaney felt that he was in a much stronger position for the election and so he should have been, having spent thousands of pounds on the campaign.

This system of election on the votes of subscribers was a carry-over from English hospitals. It was not unreasonable that "consumers" should have a say in who might be appointed to treat them, the main problem was that they had the only say. This was unfortunate for at that time they could hardly be regarded as "informed" consumers. There were no publications of hospital results and there was certainly no information available to reflect the performance of individual staff members. Systems for measuring or auditing clinical performance did not become accepted practice until the latter half of the 20th century. The nearest thing to a staff performance review then was the regular publication in the newspapers, often with lurid detail, of the findings of the many inquests into hospital deaths. In general, however, the deaths were more often considered due, and probably rightly so, to the illnesses themselves, or to causes unknown at that time, and not to inadequacies on the part of the providers of the limited care, which was then available.

This widespread election system, which lasted until 1910, resulted in canvassing. It was said, by one disgruntled staff member, that 'it was the largest purse that won the day and not a man's qualifications.' In 1891 there was a lengthy leading article in that respected English medical journal, *The Lancet,* concerning the practice of advertising by medical practitioners in Australia. It was written by the journal's Australian correspondent (unnamed), who referred, sarcastically, to the 'democratic' system of election to hospital positions in the colonies, whereby the subscribers determined the appointees. The editorial ended with an extremely severe judgement on doctors in Australia:

> Medical etiquette, as understood in Great Britain and Ireland, is unknown here. The one and only aim is to become rich, and in the pursuit of wealth most of the kindly and honourable feelings which have characterised the profession and made it noble, are trodden underfoot.

An earlier comment in the same editorial was

> The Melbourne medical men are perhaps the greatest adepts at blowing their own trumpets.

The extraordinary "honorary" staff system, that is, appointments without remuneration, was also a carry over from England and was to last for another hundred years. The "best" medical specialists were expected to earn their income from their private patients and to treat the "indigent" in the hospital for free. The teaching of medical students in the clinical or hospital part of the medical course (i.e. around the bedside), that began at the Melbourne Hospital with just three students in 1864, was likewise generally performed without remuneration, and the students' welcome to the hospital was "lukewarm". Only the teachers in the pre-clinical years and those clinicians, who were formally appointed as lecturers, were paid. Despite this apparent "ad hoc" system of teaching, the resulting graduates were considered to be capable doctors.

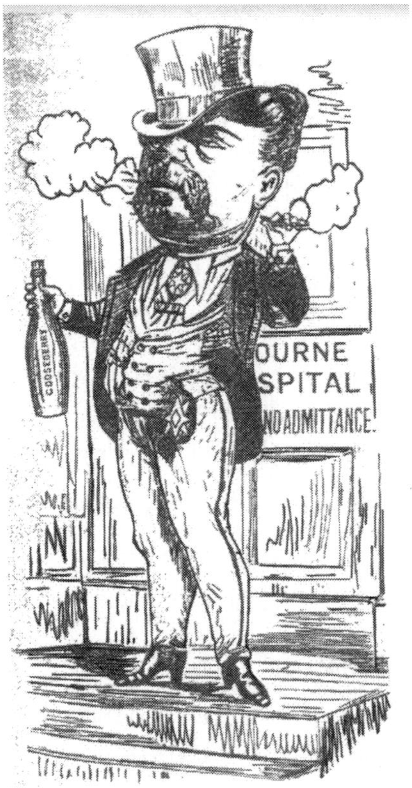

Figure 3: Caricature of 'Champagne' Jimmy

In 1875 James George Beaney was in his late 40s. He was short in stature, with a podgy build and was said to have a squeaky voice, for which he had numerous elocution lessons to enhance his appeal as a public speaker. His hair was parted in the middle and rose up on each side of the part, almost as an extension of his ears. In keeping with the fashion, he had a large drooping moustache and a small beard. Except for his pale blue eyes, referred to by some who did not regard him kindly as "shifty", an observer might have got the impression of a small bull. Indeed cartoonists in several Melbourne papers often had a field day with 'Diamond Jim' Beaney. Not surprisingly they had never come across such an ostentatious surgeon and he was frequently caricatured. Apparently Beaney did not react unfavourably to such portrayals, presumably on the basis that he would be all the better known in the community. Thus, like some current day politicians and prominent sportsmen, as well as having a large number of detractors, he had his supporters and even some admirers.

Confusion remains about so many aspects of this man, no less than about his true birth date. The most reliable source suggests that he was born in Canterbury, Kent, on 15 January 1828, but in an obituary in *The Australian Medical Gazette* in July 1891 his year of birth is given as 1831 and the date of his death on his Melbourne Cemetery monument is 30 June 1891, with his age as 59 years, which would suggest that he was born in 1832. The records in Kent prior to 1837 are scant and the confusion is further added to by the possibility that his father's surname was Beney and the 'a' was added later by James Beaney himself. Nevertheless it is clear that he was born into a fairly poor family in the Northgate area of Canterbury. His father died within a year or two of his birth, leaving his then pregnant mother to bring up James and his older brother George, and to keep the family out of the workhouse by engaging as a shoe-binder, stitching leather. It is likely that these early experiences influenced Beaney to make a better life for himself.

By 1875 he had done so having become a very busy surgeon. His income was reported to be the highest of any doctor in the colony, at between £12000 and £14,000 per annum. This was when the yearly wage of a labourer in Melbourne was just £100 and that of a skilled worker £400.

It was claimed that Beaney often requested payment in advance, and that his advice to patients on their "parlous state", which needed to be remedied by surgery "without delay" was frequently exaggerated. However he would not have been alone in this practice and from my years in surgery I am certainly aware of the occasional surgeon who has told a patient that he/she had come "just in time". There was probably also quite a degree of envy by Beaney's medical colleagues because he flaunted his financial success. He wore diamond and ruby rings on his fingers and a bejewelled gold fob watch and chain in his always colourful vest. The jewellery he wore was estimated to be worth in excess of £10,000. The implication was "he must be a good doctor because he has so much money" just as an address in Collins Street in later years carried the same reassuring implication "Ah! He's a Collins Street Specialist".

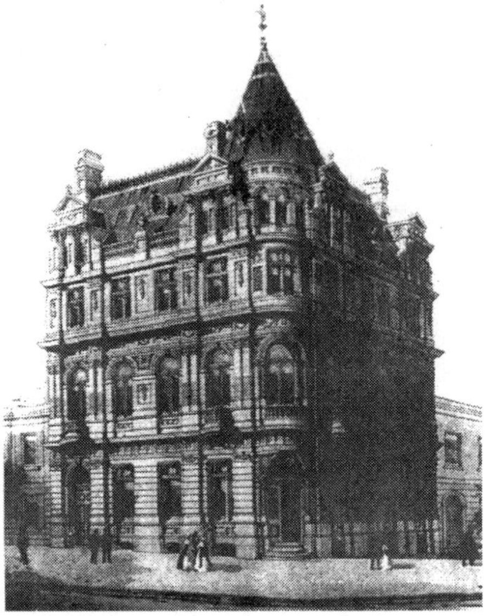

Figure 4: Cromwell House.

Not long after his hospital reappointment Beaney contracted with an architect, William Salway, to design a new house. Salway was by then well known in Melbourne as he had designed the ornate twin towered Australian Church, which stood in Flinders Street until the 1980s, impressive grandstands at the Melbourne Cricket Ground and the Caulfield racecourse, and mansions such as Raheen in Studley Park Road, Kew, which was later to become the home of Archbishop Daniel Mannix for many years, until following his death it was sold to a businessman, the late Richard Pratt. A massive four-story mansion was planned for Dr. Beaney. It was to be sited on the southeast corner of Collins and Russell streets, in the "Paris end" of Collins Street, as it was becoming known in Melbourne, and the house was to be built in a "conservative" Renaissance style.

That eastern end of Collins Street should really have been called the Roman end as most of the new buildings had an ornate Italian design. Beaney's mansion, later named Cromwell House, when completed would serve first and foremost as a residence, with ample domiciliary and entertaining areas, including a roof garden with wrought iron surrounds. It would also contain his consulting room, a separate examination area and, later, a small operating theatre and rooms for patient accommodation. The ornate building remains today with the large Hyatt on Collins Hotel towering behind it.

James Beaney had weathered two ghastly trials held nine years beforehand. They had concerned the death of a young woman, Mary Lewis, described as a pretty twenty-one-year-old barmaid, who had worked and resided at the Terminus Hotel in St. Kilda. The Terminus Hotel was situated in Fitzroy Street opposite the St Kilda railway terminus. It was a well-respected place to stay long and short term for the many visitors to the beachside suburb, and it was well located for those who came to St Kilda by rail. Although the distance from the centre of the city was less than four miles (seven kilometres) there was still some trepidation, when the Terminus Hotel was built in 1857, about travelling by road in case of a misadventure, as pictured famously by the artist William Strutt in his *Bushrangers on St Kilda Road.* The actual railway station building remains and as such is the oldest railway building in the State, but the Terminus Hotel was replaced by the more elegant looking George Hotel in the 1880s.

Mary Lewis had died following a rupture of the uterus and Beaney was charged with carrying out an abortion and causing her death. As Dr. James Rudall, the Melbourne Hospital's pathologist at the time, in a gross oversight, had thrown out the deceased's ovaries after the postmortem, the Crown Prosecutor could not prove, in the absence of evidence of changes consistent with pregnancy in one of the ovaries, that Mary Lewis had been pregnant. He could not therefore establish a reason for Beaney to have performed a curettage when he visited her at the hotel or when she consulted him at his surgery, a few days before her death.

The first trial, in the Supreme Court, lasted eleven harrowing days, at the end of which the jury had disagreed. They may have been somewhat confused by the judge, Sir Redmond Barry, who went through the whole history of the case in tedious detail, including all of the various conflicting theories presented. However he subsequently directed them to let their verdict be based upon the proven facts and not be influenced by those theories. This proved difficult for the all-male jury. The policeman assigned to the Lewis case, Inspector John Sadleir, claimed afterwards that Beaney had escaped from that first trial by only one vote. Sadleir would later be at the scene of the bushranger Ned Kelly's capture. Like Kelly he was an excellent horseman with a good knowledge of the bush and, because of these skills, he had some years earlier offered to accompany his friend Robert O'Hara Burke on his disastrous 1860 expedition to the north, with Wills. Fortunately for Sadleir, Burke declined the offer, citing Sadleir's own family commitments, for he had twelve children. At the siege of Glenrowan, Sadleir was the Superintendent in charge of the police contingent and it was he, with a constable Hugh Bracken, who prevented a police sergeant from shooting the wounded Ned Kelly dead at the end of the siege. Sadleir was one of nine recipients who shared the £8,000 reward for the capture of the Kelly Gang, his portion being just over £240.

Beaney had to then face a retrial some months later and it was seriously rumoured that if he was found guilty this time he would hang! Indeed it might have been so but for the brilliance of Butler Cole Aspinall, his defending barrister, who destroyed the credibility of Rudall and other witnesses. Some six years beforehand Aspinall, an Englishman, had made his name defending (free of charge) the gold-mining rebels from the Eureka Stockade. Thirteen diggers were brought to trial. In the first case Aspinall appeared before Chief Justice William à Beckett and to the delight of the people of Melbourne and Ballarat he managed to have the first "digger", an African-American called John Joseph, acquitted. John Joseph was apparently carried around the streets of

Melbourne triumphantly in a chair until late into the night. Subsequently all of the remaining twelve accused men were acquitted before Justice Redmond Barry.

Aspinall's performance in Beaney's re-trial certainly impressed Justice Edward E. Williams. As he had done in the first trial, the pathologist, Dr. Rudall, gave evidence. Rudall had been well trained in medicine at St. Thomas's Hospital in London and had obtained his FRCS in 1857. However, he had been in the colony only a short time and had just begun performing autopsies for the Coroner to supplement his income whilst trying to build up his practice.

He would later obtain an appointment as a general and eye surgeon at the Alfred Hospital, where his fastidious habits extended to wearing an apron, with pockets, over his usual operating coat. He kept his own instruments in these pockets, into which, incredible as it sounds now, they were swiftly returned after each one was used and only "cleaned" at the end of the day's operating. He was a small man with bristling sandy hair and a beard and, because of his irritability, some in the hospital likened him to a nervous terrier.

At the retrial Rudall didn't have the confidence of the tall and handsome Aspinall, whose command of English and sharp wit proved to be a powerful combination. The judge commended Aspinall for not calling any defence witnesses, presumably for shortening the duration of the trial, and his summing up was clearly in favour of Beaney. Critics of Justice Williams said that he was 'less able and industrious' than his colleagues and it was recognised that he seldom occupied the Court's time with long dissertations. However general opinion was that such criticism was unfair and that he was committed to his work but was simply not as colourful as contemporaries such as Barry. The jury acquitted Dr. Beaney after only ten minutes deliberation. The verdict was said to have occasioned uproarious applause in the court. It would not be the last time the skills of a barrister were required to save Beaney's "bacon".

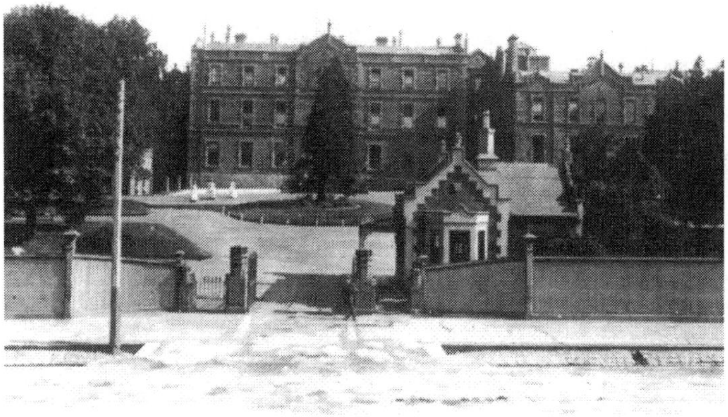

Figure 5: Melbourne Hospital, circa 1880.

Aspinall later entered politics and was at one time the 'most sought-after dinner guest in Melbourne'. Unfortunately he was considered to have led a life of gay dissipation, which prevented him achieving the influence his talents deserved. In 1871 he had a breakdown, which ended his career. On recovery he returned to England and died in April 1875. Thus he was not there to represent Dr. Beaney at the inquest held later that same year. In an odd coincidence Aspinall's wife died just one week later than her husband, in Melbourne, and virtually penniless. However one of their six children, Butler (Cole) Aspinall, with support from relatives, was subsequently educated in England and became a prominent King's Counsel.

Another person to whom Beaney was grateful in this particular trial was his friend and colleague Dr. G. Figg, who had given evidence supportive of him. Figg was a Scottish immigrant and had a practice in Williamstown in the 1860s. He was a complex and rather hotheaded individual, who was frequently involved in legal controversy, but never actually charged with malpractice. Figg stated at the trial that his own experience extended to seven thousand midwifery cases and he believed that 'he had manipulated the uterus more than any man in Europe.'. He testified that in the case of Mary Lewis the rupture of the uterus had occurred after death and that both Dr. Rudall and a Dr. William Pugh, who assisted at the post-mortem, had conducted a careless examination. Beaney later rewarded Dr. Figg with a huge silver cup at a celebratory dinner. Dr. Figg's claims of immense clinical skills and vast experience were highly unlikely to be true as a decade later Dr. Figg was asked by the Board of Health to resign on the grounds of incompetence and inefficiency. His qualifications had apparently been questioned previously, whereas the qualifications of Rudall and Pugh, also a surgeon, whom Figg had so strongly criticised, were beyond doubt.

It had certainly been a long, gruelling and very public experience for James Beaney, during one stage of which demonstrators, who had gathered outside his house, threw stones at him. On another occasion when a demonstrator actually entered his home, red faced and in a high rage, Beaney coolly suggested to the intruder that he calm down and have a drink or his blood pressure would kill him. The unsavoury publicity surrounding the trials was most likely the reason Beaney had lost his hospital appointment, but it did not reduce his flamboyance.

The Melbourne Hospital, at that time, was on the corner of Swanston and Lonsdale Streets. Patients could access it by a horse-drawn tram running along Swanston Street. This 'Broadway stage', as it had come to be called, was introduced into Melbourne from America by Francis Clapp in 1869. Behind the large iron gates of the hospital a gravel path led up around a circular lawn, to the hospital buildings, which were set well back from the street. It was later to be known as the Queen Victoria Hospital. When the 'Queen Vic' moved east in 1987 to become the Monash Medical Centre at Clayton only the central tower of the old hospital was retained. The tower did not exist in Beaney's time, however, as it dates only from 1910.

There was little to lift the spirits of the unfortunate patients who entered the Melbourne Hospital, or any other one, in Victorian times. Whilst some of today's older health carers might sigh nostalgically for the long and open "Nightingale" wards, the actual ones were sombre and austere, and the suffering of any one patient was shared by all. Around one in five patients would not survive, death being very often due to infection, possibly acquired in the hospital. Despite community concern that the hospital was a house of sepsis, Beaney knew that regaining an appointment at the Melbourne Hospital would further consolidate his surgical reputation.

The announcement of hospital appointments in 1875 was, as customary, a very public occasion. The committee room was rearranged for the announcement of the election results and members of the press were invited. Edward Cohen, the honorary treasurer and effectively the chairman of the hospital for the previous twenty odd years, presented a brief report on the year's progress. Cohen had been the Mayor of Melbourne in 1862 and was currently a Member of Parliament as well as a Director and Chairman of the Colonial Bank having been, after his arrival from England, an auctioneer and then a tea merchant. His assets included a large sheep station on the Murray River, as well as property in Melbourne. Cohen was only 54 when he died in 1877, being survived by his wife and eight children, to whom he left an estate of £29,000.

On that morning in 1875 he told the meeting that at that stage of the year the hospital looked like equalling or exceeding the previous year's record of treating over three and a half thousand in-patients and over twenty thousand outpatients. On the financial side, although the annual government grant remained low at not much over £15,000, the hospital had done well that year from the "Hospital Sunday" collection, receiving over £3,300.

Cohen then moved to the main interest of the morning, the election of the medical staff. There were no surprises with the physicians, who were announced first, except that Patrick Moloney, a young Melbourne graduate, topped the physician's poll. Then came the announcement of the surgical appointments. It would have been to his immense pleasure that Beaney heard his name read out first, with over fourteen hundred votes, followed by Fitzgerald, James and Howett. Drs. Barker and Rudall were "retired". Many of the hospital staff then present regarded these retirements as disappointing and as an embarrassment to the hospital, given their previous conscientious service.

James Beaney and his wife Mary entertained a small group of friends well that evening in the Crystal Bar at the Theatre Royal in Bourke Street, before the program commenced and during the interval. The group included his publisher Baillière, David McArthur his banker, known affectionately by those who had been recipients of his generous loans, as 'The Squire from the Heidelberg Hills', McArthur's wife Elizabeth and Dr. John Webb and his young wife. Webb had also been elected to the hospital that morning as Assistant Surgeon and, although somewhat in awe of Beaney, would have been delighted to receive the invitation to celebrate with his senior colleague. Madame Fanny Janauschek from America, who was performing that night at the Royal in *Chesney Wold,* a drama adapted from the novel *Bleak House* by Charles Dickens, accepted Beaney's invitation to join them for supper after the show.

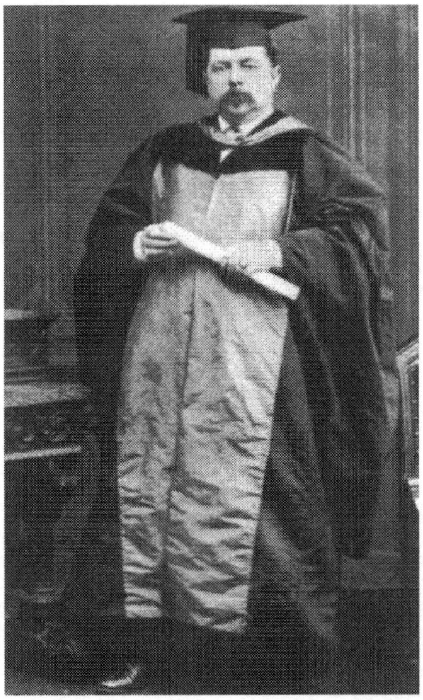

Figure 6: Dr. Beaney in his academic gown.

Fanny Janauschek was born in Prague in 1829 and went to America at the age of 38, speaking only German. However within three years she had mastered sufficient English to appear on the stage and become famous as a Shakespearean actress. Like many other world-acclaimed actors and actresses (then a politically correct term) at that time she was attracted to the theatres of the great southern city of Melbourne.

2. Settling back into the hospital

The weeks that followed Beaney's re-election to the hospital were busy ones. He had some difficulty readjusting the routines of his private practice to allow time for his hospital duties, which consisted of ward rounds and operating. The ward rounds took longer than he recalled as there were now students to teach. However, unlike some of his colleagues and being quite a showman, he enjoyed these immensely. Even the honorary surgeon, Thomas Fitzgerald, apparently recognised his enthusiasm for teaching, although Fitzgerald was known to be critical of Beaney's sweeping statements and claims of success for operations without proof. In contrast to Beaney, Fitzgerald was not a gifted lecturer but taught by example at the bedside and through his dexterity in the operating room. He was the surgeon for whom most of the junior staff wished to work, and he was said to have the 'tactus eruditis'.[1] He would later be knighted, the first Australian to be so honoured for eminence in the medical profession.

Beaney, on the other hand, endeared himself to the students as an extrovert, not only through his colourful

---

1 a sensitive touch acquired by long practice

appearance but also with his anecdotes. His ward rounds were interspersed with stories of his experiences in the Crimean War. He claimed to have won a medal as a coopted member of a Turkish Regiment, but to his critics this remained a doubtful event. Rumour had it that it was the equivalent of a two-shilling piece, given to him by a Turkish Sultan. It is also likely that his time in the Lancashire Infantry Regiment was spent in Gibraltar and that he only reached the Crimea when the war was over.

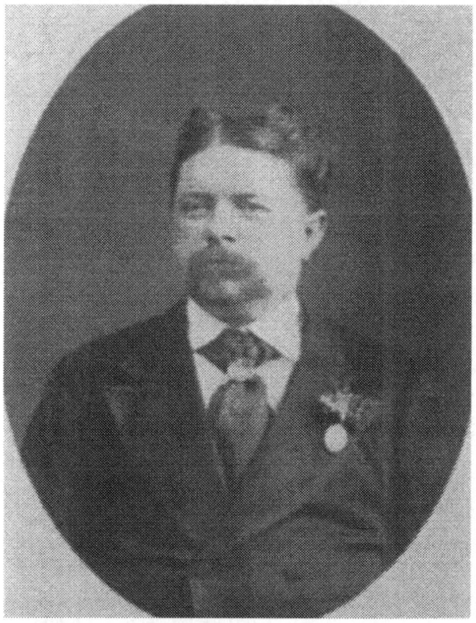

Figure 7: Dr. Beaney, wearing his Crimea medal.

Beaney also recounted stories from the seamy parts of Paris where he studied venereology, and shared some humorous experiences. He told the students he had encountered as an assistant in a chemist shop in Collins Street, a position he said he obtained when he first arrived in the Colony. He had also worked in a chemist shop in Canterbury as a teenager, before working as an errand boy for a local doctor. His enthusiasm was recognised by that doctor and his next step up was to be apprenticed to a surgeon, William Cooper, a brother of Thomas Sidney Cooper, the noted English landscape artist. William Cooper encouraged the young Beaney to undertake medical studies, which he did. However in his early twenties, whilst in medical school, he became quite ill. He blamed this on "hard work" and he was advised to take a long sea voyage. He almost certainly had tuberculosis, which was at that time known as consumption or phthisis. It was regarded in the early part of the 19th century as an hereditary constitutional disease rather than a contagious one and was recognised as a sign of poverty as well as being an unfortunate and unavoidable part of the industrialised world. Around 40% of working-class deaths in that period were due to tuberculosis.

Beaney travelled to America before arriving in Melbourne in 1852. There he lodged with the Honourable John Wood, MLC, who ran a pharmacy and he was obliged to work in it. It is likely that all he did there was wash bottles and pound pills as payment for his lodging. A year or two later he returned to England and in 1855 obtained a diploma in surgery in Edinburgh. It was said of diplomas given at that time, probably unfairly, that with the shortage of surgeons during the Crimean War the examination became notoriously lax. Beaney returned to Melbourne in 1858 and became an assistant to Dr. John Maund, in a thriving Collins Street practice, to which he succeeded when Dr. Maund died less than a year later. Two years before he died Dr. Maund had aided Frances Perry, the wife of the Anglican Bishop of Melbourne, in establishing the Melbourne Lying-in Hospital, which would later become the Royal Women's Hospital.

In 1860 Beaney was awarded a Fellowship of Surgery (FRCS) from the Royal College of Surgeons, Edinburgh, and in that same year was appointed, for the first time, as a surgeon to the Melbourne Hospital, the Fellowship being recognised as a specialist qualification.

Beaney would have endeared himself even more to medical students and to the University authorities when, several years later, he established the Beaney prizes for the top students. The prizes exist to this day as scholarships (as indicated above) but are not surrounded by the ceremony Beaney established for them. Such was his influence that he persuaded the top men of science in the colony to deliver eloquent addresses and then to present the Beaney medals, generally in the presence of the press.

There had been considerable friction between the Melbourne Hospital and the new Medical School even before the latter commenced functioning officially in 1862. The first issue was concerned with its location, with there being a disagreement as to whether it should be at the University in Carlton, or in the city adjacent to the hospital. A second major issue was, from the University's point of view, the lack of influence it had over who might lecture the students, for it had no say in the appointment of the medical staff to the Melbourne Hospital. For example, the first lecturer in surgery, Dr. Edward Barker, did not have a hospital appointment when he commenced as a University lecturer.

For nearly three decades the University was to continually express its disappointment at the attitude of the honorary medical staff at the hospital with regard to student teaching. Many of the honorary staff members were lax in their attendance to deliver lectures promised and some were even hostile to the students. It was not until 1884 that "clinical" teachers were officially appointed. The first appointments were Dr. John Williams in medicine and Mr. Thomas Fitzgerald in surgery. However, once they were appointed, the other members of the honorary staff (Beaney excluded) determined that they would not give any lectures, although they were still prepared to divide the more than £500 provided in students lecture fees amongst themselves.

It wasn't until the early 1900s that the University was able to influence appointments to hospital staff through the establishment of Hospital Advisory Boards, which included University representatives.

As with the honorary medical staff the student community was entirely male, the first female students not being admitted to the faculty until 1887. Five years later a female student, Margaret Whyte, was to "top" the year in medicine and surgery. There was great argument initially as to whether teaching of the female medical students should be separate from the males. Fortunately commonsense prevailed in the pre-clinical teaching, but for some years the clinical teaching of the female medical students, around the patient's bed, was done separately down on the other side of the river at the Alfred Hospital, which had been functioning since 1871.

In addition to student teaching, Beaney also enjoyed teaching the resident staff and many an operating session would be followed, at the end of the day, by further informal tutoring over a glass or more of champagne, a supply of which he apparently kept in his carriage, parked in the hospital grounds. It was a Hansom cab, a light single horse-drawn vehicle that had been designed by Joseph Hansom in York in 1834 and which, like Henry Ford's T model early in the 20th century, rapidly swept the world. Fergus Hulme's novel *The mystery of a Hansom Cab,* which was set in Melbourne, also swept the world when it was published in 1886, outselling Arthur Conan Doyle's first Sherlock Holmes novel *A Study in Scarlet.* Hulme's novel certainly gave the outside world some idea of Melbourne's varied social life in that era.

Beaney's manner with patients was apparently not unkind, or at least was never reported as such. He was generous in his prescription of brandy, and frequently champagne as well, to ease their suffering. Some staff, including the hospital accountant, with knowledge of the hospital expenditure on alcohol, considered him overgenerous in this practice. Beaney was not alone however in prescribing alcohol as there were few other effective medications available to the profession, in the practice of Western medicine before the turn of the century, except perhaps for the Birmingham physician Withering's foxglove extract (now known as digitalis), which had been used since the previous century for disorders of the heart.

Alcohol was certainly also prevalent in the Melbourne community. There were over one thousand "public" houses in the city, with around one hundred each in the inner suburbs of Fitzroy and Collingwood alone. In the latter suburb there were six breweries and two distilleries. Their tall brewing stacks were said to rival the church spires of the more affluent suburbs.

The grimness of the surgical problems encountered at that time is illustrated by the case of an otherwise healthy twenty-eight-year-old man whose right leg was run over by the carriage of a shunting train, when his foot was caught in a crossing. He suffered a compound (open) fracture of the leg with multiple bone fragments visible in a gaping wound. Three days following admission to the Melbourne Hospital he became delirious, as infection set in. Despite Beaney's efforts to cleanse the wound and realign the bones, gangrene resulted. The patient refused an amputation and all Beaney could prescribe was alcohol to ease his pain and keep him oblivious of the circumstances until death followed some two and a half weeks later.

It was no wonder that the water from the little grotto of Lourdes, in the Pyrenees, had become so sought after by patients or their relatives over the previous fifteen years, in the hope of achieving a miracle cure. The "germ" theory was ill understood and few surgeons in the colony, including Beaney, even if they were aware of the concept, followed Professor Joseph Lister's principles of antisepsis, as they were regarded as complex and time consuming to apply.

"Listerism", as it came to be called, initially involved the use of creosote dressings for wounds and later the use of a carbolic spray passing over the operating field. It was further extended to the use of gloves by the operator and to the frequent washing in 5% carbolic acid solution. In 1867, in the medical journal, *The Lancet,* Lister published the results of his treatment in this manner for eleven cases of lower limb compound fractures, similar to Beaney's case, with the avoidance of gangrene in all. Bone union was subsequently achieved in nine of the eleven patients, a result unheard of before then.

If the colonial surgeons were slow to "pick up" on his techniques, they were not alone. It seems extraordinary to us now, but even prominent surgeons such as London's Watson Cheyene, Lawson Tait in Birmingham and the great Samuel Gross in Philadelphia ridiculed Lister and the work he performed in Scotland. The first use of his principles in the colonies was by Dr. S. Hogarth Pringle (who was an intern with Lister) late in 1867 in New South Wales and by Dr. William Gilbee (an ex-gold digger) at the Melbourne Hospital, towards the end of the same year.

The value of Listerism was still being argued a decade later, in the *Australian Medical Journal* and for even longer in *The Lancet.* The publication of a series of successful cases of primary healing by Dr. Thorpe Girdlestone, from the Melbourne Hospital in 1887, ensured that the majority of the colony's surgeons, from then on, would adhere to principles of antisepsis. After the turn of the century antisepsis gave way to striving for cleanliness or "asepsis". Another of Girdlestone's claims to fame, incidentally, was the use of kangaroo tendon as a suture material. It did not however replace the more popular and more readily available horsehair. It was interesting that Thomas Fitzgerald, whilst lacking the biological insight of Lister, had appreciated the significant difference in outcomes between simple and open or compound fractures and had designed a whole series of subcutaneous operations to avoid the as yet unexplained complications of infection. For a totally different and unclear reason he had introduced a concept of what is known today as "keyhole" surgery.

Rather than accept that infection was from direct contact with germs it was easier, in 1875, to believe in the "miasmic" or airborne theory of infection. The air in many of the city's inner areas, such as

Collingwood, was grossly polluted by open sewage, tannery fumes and slaughterhouse refuse. It was odd that Melbourne should have been so far in advance of other cities with its abundant supply of uncontaminated water, which had been coming from the Yan Yean Reservoir since 1857, yet so far behind in its limited ability to cope with its sewage. Much of its sewage ended up in the Yarra River, earning Melbourne the nicknames, from its Sydney rivals, of "Smell boom"and "Smellbourne".

Sewage was not the only waste material that ended up in the Yarra. In the industrial suburb of Collingwood, which was rapidly becoming the 'Manchester of the South', the noxious waste from the factories was emptied into it. Many of the traders, who owned those factories, were also local councillors and were able to win repeal of the Yarra pollution laws. The state of the river slowly worsened as the volume and rate of production of locally made goods increased.

Arthur Snowdon, a city lawyer, was one of very few to speak against pollution at Collingwood council meetings. Like so many young Englishmen he was attracted to the Victorian goldfields, but after two unsuccessful years went to Melbourne and obtained a position as a law clerk, subsequently graduating in law. He was later Mayor of Melbourne for three terms and received a knighthood, but he had limited success in his attempts to reduce pollution in the swampy Collingwood flatlands.

In addition to disinterest from the manufacturers of Melbourne, it may also have been a matter of there being no public works money left for a sewage system, as the Yan Yean water project had been very costly. Over 400 workers had been employed in a diversion of water to Melbourne from the north-east Plenty River and when the main valve was turned on in the Carlton Gardens in 1857, the cost of the project was estimated at around £750,000, which was a quite considerable over-run. It would not be until the 1890s, after years of argument, that Melbourne was sewered. The Yan Yean Reservoir was taken off-line in 2007, after providing water to the City of Melbourne for 150 years. Remnants of that system can still be seen along the central strip in St Georges Road, Northcote.

3. 1875 Melbourne: more and less marvellous

Due to the many millions of pounds worth of gold coming into the city from the mid-Victorian gold fields, Melbourne, by 1875, had become one of the richest cities in the world. It had been named Melbourne in 1837 by Sir Richard Bourke, the Governor of New South Wales, after William Lamb, the second Viscount Melbourne, who was Prime Minister of England when Queen Victoria came to the throne, so the name was apt for the colony bearing her name. However the region was known as the Port Phillip District and was not called Victoria until 1851, through a British Act of Parliament that separated it from New South Wales. Some doubt exists as to whether Lord Melbourne was really the son of his mother's husband, but that did not prove a hindrance to his successful political career, nor did the affair his wife Lady Caroline (née Ponsonby) had with Lord Byron, although when the affair finally became public he separated from her. He was of great assistance to the young Queen Victoria, who publicly acknowledged his guidance in the early years of her reign.

The city's planners, prominent amongst whom was Sir Redmond Barry, had early on embarked upon a massive program of building to enhance Melbourne's stature as a sophisticated city. Barry, an Irishman and a bachelor, had been appointed a Supreme Court judge in 1852 and was knighted in 1860. He was a co-founder of Melbourne University and its first Chancellor. He was also instrumental in the development of the Public Library. He maintained an excellent library in his own house, which later became part of the "old" Children's Hospital in Carlton. One thing he had in common with Beaney was a love of wine. Barry was a connoisseur and dispersed hospitality to the "notables" of the day, with some sophistication. When he entertained, he would appear in a blue tailcoat with large gilt buttons, silk breeches, stockings, and buckled shoes. The opening of each vintage bottle was usually preceded by a short poem eulogising its special characteristics. However, Barry's name was to live on in later years, as much for his role as the judge in the 1880 trial of the bushranger, Ned Kelly, as it would for his grand cultural achievements. Kelly had a great many sympathisers in the Irish community of mid and northern Victoria and to these, and other observers, it seemed that Barry rushed Kelly's trial and that not all of the available evidence was properly heard. Rumour was that he had a function to attend at Government House and hated to offend the Vice-Regal personage by a late arrival. Following Barry's pronouncement of the death sentence upon Kelly and the 'May God have mercy on your soul', Ned prophesied that Barry would join him very soon, and he did. Ned Kelly was hanged on the 11th November 1880. Redmond Barry fell ill two days later and he died on the 23rd November.

The Melbourne in which he had arrived in 1839, as a 26 years old lawyer, was a "wild west" village compared with the significant city he helped establish, with its grand buildings and boulevards, at the time of his death at the age of 67. His statue stands in Swanston Street outside the Public Library, one block away from the Old Melbourne Gaol, where Kelly was hanged. His gravestone in the Melbourne Cemetery did not mention that buried with him is Louisa Barrow, his beloved mistress and the mother of the four children who bore his name. Their existence had not been disclosed in the Victorian era. However 130 years later the Melbourne General Cemetery erected a plaque to mark the presence of Louise Barrow's body there.

Those city planners capitalised on the wide streets and the ample parks, which had been set out with remarkable forethought by Robert Hoddle in 1837. By the mid 1870s the city area also had many elaborate two, three and four storey high buildings lining its wide streets and bordering the parks. A number of them such as the Melbourne Town Hall, the Public Library, the General Post Office and the Treasury had a classic Italian architecture. This was popular in England at the time and it was considered that it suited the climate of the southern colony.

The Treasury building was amongst the finest of these structures. It sat at the top of the eastern end of Collins Street facing west. Amazingly a Mr. J.J. Clarke designed it when he was a nineteen-year-old draftsman in the Public Works Department. It was his first major work and resembled Sansovino's Villa Garzoni in Northern Italy, with its elegant edifice. The Royal Mint was another, built to resemble a palace designed by Donato Bramante, who had introduced Italy to the Renaissance style with its domes, columns and arches, all of minimal depth on a virtually flat wall. Bramante drew up the original design, subsequently developed further by Michelangelo, for St Peter's Basilica in Rome.

By 1875 the magnificent Supreme Court building was almost finished and work had begun on the Exhibition Building, which was to hold a great international exhibition in 1880 (and another one in 1888 to mark the centenary of colonisation). The exhibition was the brainchild of the politician Graham Berry, the champion of the "working classes", who wished to show the world what Melbourne could manufacture. The cost of the building was to be £250,000, which was regarded by Redmond Barry as far too extravagant, and he resigned from the Committee of Management. The Exhibition in 1880, however, was an overwhelming success, the building itself being another one with an Italian basis, being modelled on Brunelleschi's cathedral in Florence.

The city abounded in architects, plasterers (many skilled Italians were especially brought out to Melbourne), and other artisans such as tilers, bricklayers and painters. They all contributed to the prodigious growth of the city that in 1885 would be dubbed by the English journalist, George Sala, 'Marvellous Melbourne'.

George Augustus Sala, or GAS as he liked to sign his articles, was regarded as the "Prince" of English journalists. He was a fairly pompous fellow with a well-rounded figure and a classical drooping moustache. Having been forewarned of his coming to Melbourne a number of the city "fathers" ensured that he was well accommodated at Scotts Hotel in Collins Street and called upon him to offer their assistance during his visit. The visit was a great success except for two things. A minor one was that he received sharp criticism, which became public, from the members of the Yorick Club for declining their invitation to dinner at the club. The membership of that club was composed mainly of "literary" men, i.e. journalists like Sara. Presumably Dr. Beaney, who was also a member, regarded himself as a literary man in view of his many medical publications. The Yorick Club was absorbed into the Savage Club, which still exists, in the following century. On a much sadder note Sara's wife, Harriet died on that visit to Melbourne and she was buried in the Melbourne Cemetery, Sara returning to England alone.

The Fitzroy Gardens and Royal Botanic Gardens had already been established and grand houses of worship erected in the city and inner suburbs. All of these further added to a sought after air of dignity, confirming that the city was not only a financial and trading metropolis but also one possessed of a quality of living (for some of the population) equal to that in any European city.

Many of the magnificent homes that were springing up in the suburbs also had an Italian style and were accordingly named; for example, Como, Mentone and Leura. Fine terraces, such as Royal Terrace in Fitzroy and Burlington Terrace in East Melbourne, were built on the edge of the city to house the businessmen of the time.

Anthony Trollope, the noted English novelist, had visited Melbourne in 1871 and marvelled at how well the workingman or artisan could do for himself – 'perhaps better than anywhere else in the world'. On the down side he found many Australians to be boastful and Melburnians in this respect the worst 'braggarts' of all. These comments were included in a book *Australia and New Zealand,* which he wrote after his visit and the Australian papers were quite hostile to the criticism. It is likely that this prolific author, best known for his *Chronicles of Barsetshire,* remained highly sensitive to human interaction through his unhappy childhood experiences of severe and persistent bullying. A lesser-known fact about Trollope is that for most of his working life he held executive positions within the English postal system and is attributed with introducing the iconic red pillar-boxes.

A number of the successful doctors of the day established large stylish homes in Collins Street and practiced from those homes, as did Beaney. His

Cromwell House, when finished, was four stories high and capped by a wrought iron fence around a roof garden with a tower on the front corner. The tower was supposedly built to rival the one on Scots Church, which stood diagonally opposite on the northwest corner. Another Melbourne Hospital surgeon, Edwin James, lived in the very large Alcaston House on the corner of Collins and Spring Street. It stood until 1929, when it was replaced with a seven story building in a mixed Renaissance and modern design, which blended well with the Treasury area. The physician Dr. John Williams lived in another large Renaissance house at 70 Collins Street and Dr. Aubrey Brown and his wife lived in 8 Portland Place, Collins Street. Few of them, however, would have matched Beaney in the lavishness of his home entertainment.

Beaney was probably around forty-two years old when he married Susannah Mary Griffiths in Wales. They had no children. Beaney, perhaps more than his wife, enjoyed and even sought the social life available to them. It is likely that he encouraged her to be outfitted, as he was, by the drapers W.H. and A.H. George, mostly in velvet and pure linen. A.H. George had trained in the leading fashion houses of London and Paris and the brothers were not in business long before they moved their drapery shop from Collingwood to Collins Street, initially in a central part of the city, before moving towards the "Paris" end and becoming the department store for the elite. Trading in the iconic building, which still stands, continued until 1995. A very good suit in the 1870s could be obtained for less than five pounds. Other comparative prices were whiskey at one pound five shillings a gallon, milk at four pence a quart, and a lettuce for just one penny.

Large retail stores, such as Buckley and Nunn's, were already established in Bourke Street and much fine locally made merchandise could be purchased there. Irish born Mark Buckley had made his money during the early part of the gold rush and he joined with the draper, C.J. Nunn in 1862 to purchase over 160 feet of frontage in Bourke Street. He also bought 32 acres of prime land just south of the Yarra and built the mansion Beulieu, which much later became St. Catherine's School. Buckley and Nunn's emporium was taken over by David Jones Limited in the 1980s, but the name lives on in an Australian colloquialism 'You've got Buckley's', meaning no chance of achieving or winning whatever is being disputed or discussed.

Industrial growth accompanied the building splurge in Melbourne and by 1875 there were around 1500 large factories in addition to many hundreds of brickyards, sawmills, tanneries, flourmills, breweries and distilleries. However, in contrast to the grand buildings mentioned before, "spec" builders ran up thousands of cottages in the inner suburbs to house the workers for these factories. The money came from a multitude of building societies, which had been rapidly established with minimal securities and very few safeguards. Who cared, it was a time of plenty!

The colony of Victoria had almost 800,000 people in 1875. Most were in Melbourne and it seems that the artists and performers of the world came to entertain them. Amongst those who appeared were Nellie Stewart, Sarah Bernhardt, W.S. Lyster, the father of opera in Melbourne, and George Coppin the actor, who made Sorrento, south of Melbourne, such a sought after holiday venue. Many fine hotels were built, two of the best being the "new" Menzies Hotel on the corner of Williams and Bourke Streets, and Scotts Hotel in Collins Street. Two famous guests to stay at Menzies were Alexander Graham Bell, inventor of the telephone, and Herbert Hoover, the 31st President of the United States. Hoover was a mining engineer and in his 30s he worked in the gold mining areas of Western Australia, establishing with others, the Sons of Gualia Mines, which would make him a millionaire. The Gualia mines continued to function until 1963. Hoover was also known as the 'doctor of sick mines' and he was involved in the development of Broken Hill.

Samuel Clemens (Mark Twain) is said to have worked in the boiler room of Menzies "to get fit" during his time in Australia. Another man who worked his way to the top was W.C. Wilson, who started employment at Scotts as a waiter and subsequently bought the hotel. Despite his endeavours to maintain the respectability of the hotel he was not always successful in preventing the reporting in the press of disturbances at the hotel, and his own involvement in the resolution of those disturbances. It was the place for the pastoral community of Victoria to stay as well as racehorse owners and breeders. Famous visitors included W.G. Grace of cricket fame; later, it became Dame Nellie Melba's favourite hotel. Wilson sold the hotel in 1888 for £160,000. Unfortunately, like so many of Melbourne's architecturally fine buildings, it was demolished in the 1960s.

With its popular theatres and hotels "Bourke Street on Saturday night" was where and when Melburnians spent their money in the pursuit of pleasure, with little thought of tomorrow. There were up to a dozen theatres of varying sizes and décor in Bourke Street in the late 1800s, most of them having a generally elaborate and always well-stocked bar.

It was no wonder Beaney sought also to be a Member of the Legislative Council, Victoria's upper house of Parliament. The use of political power for personal gain was widespread and clearly evident at that time. It came to be known as 'log rolling' and the period Melbourne was entering into as the 'Land Boom'. Prominent amongst the boomers were Benjamin and Theodore Fink, William Baillieu, William Bruce and James Munro. The history of the times is a little confusing, however, as there were five Finks, six Kitchens, five Davies brothers and about a dozen Baillieus, all in the public eye during that time of rapid development. The Fink Building, erected on Flinders Street by Benjamin, at ten stories high, was the tallest in the country and one of the tallest in the world in the 1880s. It was destroyed by fire in 1897.

The interest rate then was very low; for example it was 2.5% in 1873, rising briefly to 4% in 1876, before falling again. Thousands of acres of suburban land were sold and resold, each time at higher prices.

The boom was lifted further by the discovery of silver in the Wimmera region of western Victoria in 1882, by a prolific grain harvest in 1885, and by wool prices, which soared to over £20 per bale. At its height in 1887 the boom saw even the banks entering into land speculation, after a review of the *Companies Act.* Bank advances to clients were in excess of 100 million pounds. Building Societies went wild as a change in Victorian legislation permitted the buying and selling of, or mortgaging of, freehold and leasehold estates. There was no thought of caution in the 1870s and 80s and who would dare to halt the pace, as the rich became richer and the city brighter and busier.

Factory workers were not altogether unprotected at this time. Union strength had grown in Melbourne following an historic meeting of stonemasons in 1856. They had met at the Belvidere Hotel in Eastern Hill, on the corner of Brunswick Street and Victoria Parade, and voted for an eight-hour working day. Their cause might have been lost had it not been for a Fitzroy medical practitioner, Dr. Thomas Embling, who as the local member of Parliament, supported them with his slogan of eight hours labour, eight hours recreation, eight hours rest. Rudyard Kipling, another famous visitor to Melbourne not long after the introduction of the "world first" eight hour day, was surprisingly very critical of this social advance. The same hotel, in my time as a student and junior medical officer, was frequented by the staff from the nearby St Vincents Hospital. Within the hospital all of the wards were given saint's names. The first Australian intensive care unit (ICU) was formed at St Vincents and the name chosen for it was St Peters ward (so many of the patients admitted to it in its early years were already close to St Peter's pearly gates). The Eastern Hill hotel, in an even more factitious and affectionate gesture by the junior medical staff, was un-officiously called 'St Augustine's ward', St Augustine in his youth having a reputation as a wayward young man. The junior staff could openly say, in front of patients, I shall meet you in St Augustine's. The hotel was later acquired by the Sisters of Charity and is no longer a hotel, as it was converted to consulting rooms, which are used by various specialist health practitioners. (A sigh for the good old days).

One of the strongest unions in the 1870s was the boot makers' union, led by its secretary William Trenwith. Trenwith had come from Tasmania, where he had been a champion boxer, and he carried that same pugilistic aggression into his negotiations. Despite a limited education he was a gifted orator and like James Beaney he enjoyed attention and applause. He wore a smart top hat and, again like Beaney, went about his business in his own Hansom cab, doing battle with such people as Hugh Thompson, a prominent city leather merchant, who himself had started as a boot maker and tanner, and by then was living in pleasant East Melbourne but was the Mayor of Collingwood.

Whilst there was obviously much that was golden in Melbourne at that time, there was also a less attractive side to life. The colony had already established twelve jails, the two largest being in Melbourne, to cope with the increasing amount of crime, and there was a huge asylum at Kew, for the mentally "challenged". The rapid influx of wealth was certainly not distributed evenly. The journalist Stanley James, who arrived from London via America in 1875, was quick to discover and write about the poor people in the 'back slums of Melbourne'. His articles appeared in the Melbourne *Argus* under the name of 'The Vagabond'. The main "show" streets had been upgraded with wooden cross bridges every fifty yards over open drains, but many of the smaller streets, even in the city proper, left much to be desired and carried with them a constant threat of infection, from the sewage, horse manure and household slops, which flowed down open drains. Even the hospital refuse was discarded into those open drains. These circumstances, as much as the opium trade, contributed to Little Bourke Street's reputation as a 'filthy den'. Thus like any other fast growing metropolis around the world Melbourne was a city of contrasts.

Less marvellous aspects of Melbourne in 1875 were the physical dangers of the open sewage system mentioned above and epidemics of infection. In that year five children and two night workers suffocated after falling into cesspits. Typhoid and scarlet fever were rampant, as they had been in New York when it rapidly grew in the early part of the 19th century. There were over 250 cases of the latter disease reported to the Victorian Board of Health in 1875, just in the month of November.

Patients had to be made of stern stuff to survive the treatment for scarlet fever, let alone the disease. Dr. William Crooke, who was on the Health Board, would treat the whole family, his routine consisting of an emetic; an aperient; quinine; champagne and finally spa water, in that order, none of which would be of any great help apart from the provision of fluid. Dr. Crooke was not exactly a paragon of virtue. He had come over from Tasmania, attracted by stories of rapid wealth. He owned a large brick factory in Collingwood East and obtained a seat on the local council to protect his interests, but escaped the polluted air of that suburb by siting his residence in the nearby more fashionable Eastern Hill.

When, in 1874, the Government proposed an infectious diseases hospital in the adjacent suburb of Fairfield the Collingwood council, although over a third of the councilors themselves ran noxious trades, objected strongly, claiming that the winds would carry contagious gases across their holdings.

The "Bust", when it came later in 1889, was sudden and severe. Many prominent speculators went bankrupt; some were jailed, or fled the country. The severity of the crisis is exemplified by the changes to the circumstances of Mark Moss, an English financier, who initially was unsuccessful on the gold fields in mid-Victoria, but compiled a fortune as a money lender and built a magnificent "castle" in Brighton called Norwood. He was estimated to be worth £500,000 in 1890 but had just £20 on his death in 1901. However Harry Moss, the youngest of his twelve children, rather than his father's money, had inherited his business skills and also amassed a fortune, which upon his death in 1960 was estimated to be around one million pounds. He bequeathed the bulk of his estate to the Royal Children's Hospital as a perpetual trust.

For some affected by the Bust their insolvency was so great that they suicided. Amongst those reported at the time was an investor named George Ford, who after stabbing himself numerous times, bled to death in Scotts Hotel. Another was William James Irvine, a mining speculator, who threw off his clothes, waded out into the Yarra River near Princes Bridge and drowned. In 1891 four of the largest banks suspended payments and in 1893 a run on the banks forced almost all to break down. Half of Melbourne was left out of work and starving. It was in that year that the Sisters of Charity established St Vincents Hospital to tend to the sick poor, the first buildings acquired being twin terraces in Victoria Parade, on the northern border between the city and Fitzroy and not too far from the disastrously placed families in Collingwood.

Many more adventurous (or desperate) citizens moved to other places, hoping to remake their fortune on the goldfields of Coolgardie in the west of Australia, or in New Zealand and South Africa. Some speculators with influence, including the Finks, were able to negotiate a 'composition of arrangement' or 'compote' and pay out their debts at a halfpenny or penny to the pound, sometimes without the public even knowing.

Such events apparently did not trouble James Beaney, however, or at least did not force him to alter his manner of living. He may have had access to investment advice from his neighbour Jane Brown's father, Henry "Money" Miller, who was a prominent banker. He owned a large building in the western end of Collins Street, which subsequently became Melbourne's first stock exchange. Miller had an adventurous spirit, which suited the times. He was once heard to tell a budding public accountant 'If you are going to cheat, do it on a large scale and burn the bally books'. Sometimes even Miller, however, underestimated the city's rapidly rising land prices as was evident when Benjamin Fink, at the height of his financial ventures, bought Miller's bank building for £65,000 and sold it on a few months later for £120,000. When much later in 1929 George Meudall, who had been made manager of the Bank of Victoria by Henry Miller, published an uninhibited autobiography in which he outlined many of the unusual financial transactions (of the Boom/Bust period) and suggested who were involved, the biography caused a major stir. James Gillespie, the chairman of the booksellers Robertson & Mullen's, himself a land-boomer, withdrew it and warned other booksellers of possible legal consequences if they stocked it.

Despite its shortcomings, on balance, Melbourne was probably more rather than less marvellous, this spirit being captured by Henry Kendall in his poem on the Melbourne International Exhibition of 1880:

> Dressed is this beautiful city– the spires of it Burn
> in the firmament stately and still

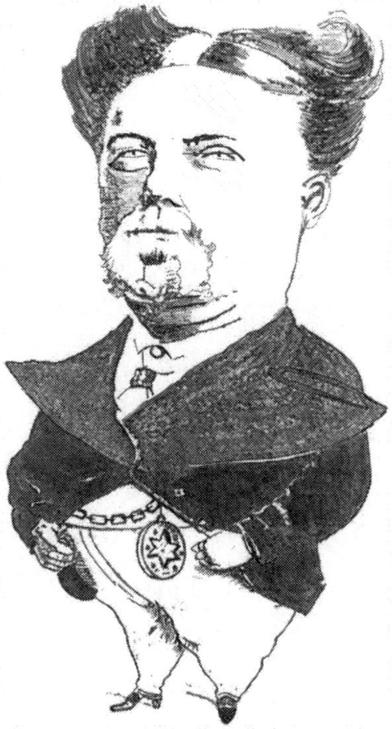

Figure 8: Caricature of 'Jelly-belly' Dr. Beaney.

4. Indulgences: pleasure, politics and a little medicine

Beaney loved fine food as well as fine wine. Being dissatisfied with the average food offered at most of the city's hotels, except perhaps for Scotts Hotel, which also had an excellent wine cellar, he joined with his jeweller friends, the Denis brothers, to form the French Club. Sylla and Victor Denis came out from France in 1853 to the Ballarat goldfields, but were unsuccessful there and moved to Melbourne, where in 1857 they established a jewellery business, which was very successful. They would, in the 1880 International Exhibition, win a First Order of Merit for gold and silver. It is likely that the jewellery, which adorned James Beaney, was purchased from the Denis brothers. It was said that dinners at the French Club, like Beaney's diamonds, were of 'the first water'. Invitations to dine with him were rarely refused.

It is not clear why Beaney was never a member of the Melbourne Club, which was so near to his house. Certainly the membership was fairly exclusive and consisted of venerable merchant bankers, squatters and a small number from the professions, with many in the club also being Members of Parliament. For Beaney there would have been no difficulty with the entrance fee of forty guineas, but perhaps the required long list of referees could not be assembled, as many people kept their distance from him.

It is interesting to note also that, although he undoubtedly enjoyed receiving attention, Beaney never sought office in either the Medical Society of Victoria or in the Victorian branch of the British Medical Association (as it was then). His name is only rarely found in the list of attendees at monthly meetings. Whether it was indicated to him that he would be unwelcome or whether he was disdainful of the Society members is not known, for at that time only around ten percent of the colony's doctors were members of the Society. Like any such professional group they were most likely composed of those with a genuine desire to improve standards, through increasing their own knowledge and also imparting it to others; those who wished to advance their careers; and those who sought power and influence (through office) to offset their own mediocre performance in the practice of their profession.

There is a record of Beaney being present, on one particular occasion, at a well-attended special meeting of the Medical Society in September 1869, called to consider the expulsion of the surgeon, Dr. Edward Barker, from the Society. At one stage there was a violent altercation between Beaney and a Dr. Richard Tracy, another Irishman who had come out to try his luck in Bendigo, with only limited success. Upon his return to Melbourne Tracy set up practice in Collins Street and, having an interest in obstetrics, he, together with Dr. Maund and Mrs. Perry, established the Melbourne Lying-in Hospital. He was the University lecturer in Obstetrics and Gynaecology at the time of this fracas with Beaney, the reason for which had been his change of attitude in midstream and his subsequent move to support Barker's retention in the Society.

The reason for the expulsion meeting is a somewhat complex story. Barker had been a support witness for a Mr. Jordan, the proprietor of the notorious Anthropological Museum, which apparently contained an inappropriate exhibition of body parts, being mainly the sexual organs. Melbourne had seen a number of such exhibitions in the previous decade, but Jordan's was apparently a particularly vulgar one. Jordan had brought a claim for defamation against *The Age,* which had vilified the Museum describing it as nothing more than a blatant display of pornography. It certainly would have been described as such today. Unfortunately Barker's support for the discredited Jordon had been reluctantly drawn from him through his having treated Jordan's wife over some years.

The Society viewed Barker's action very poorly, especially as he was, at the time, the University lecturer in surgery. At this particular meeting Barker issued an apology and a retraction of that support, in an attempt to avoid expulsion. Barker went to further pains to explain that he had returned a cheque for £21 that "Dr." Jordan had sent to help with Dr. Barker's own testimonial in a totally separate matter.

Barker's apology was accepted and the motion for his expulsion from the Society was dismissed.

Now the particular testimonial Barker referred to had been established to collect funds to reimburse him (Barker) for his expenses in another case, that of Donaldson vs. Barker, which occurred earlier that year. Donaldson, who was a patient of Barker's, had sustained a fracture of the kneecap. The treatment instigated by Barker included the application of a metal ring over the fracture. Poor supervision had lead to ischaemia of the leg, with subsequent gangrene, necessitating amputation. Donaldson sued Barker for £500 for the loss of his leg. Although Barker avoided any penalty it was made clear that, as a whole, the honorary staff of the hospital had obligations of care, by virtue of their position, which could not be passed off on to the junior staff at will.

This was a fault with many of the senior doctors. Beaney himself had once been sued (unsuccessfully) over the death of a trauma patient he failed to see despite being called no less than four times to visit the patient and advise on treatment. There were times also when he would not visit the hospital for two weeks or more. The record for non-attendance, however, was apparently held by an honorary physician, who did not set foot within the hospital grounds for six months and yet retained his position on the staff.

Beaney maintained his interest in military medicine as surgeon to the Royal Victorian Artillery and through this role established valuable city contacts such as John Templeton, manager of the National Mutual Life Association, who was also a volunteer and a Lt. Colonel in the 2nd Regiment. When the Bust came Templeton was the appointed liquidator for many of the firms in trouble, and was consequently a good friend to have on side. On account of the Russian threat (a Crimean war leftover) to Melbourne, ludicrous as it now seems, militia were formed. It was intended to establish a small volunteer corp of up to 2000 men. However this grew to 4000 by 1860 with many prominent citizens doing their duty; for example Justice Redmond Barry commanded the Fitzroy Rifles. Beaney, with his military connections, was also a co-founder of yet another club, the Pipeclay Club. This was the forerunner to the Naval and Military Club, which later boasted such distinguished members as General Sir John Monash and Field Marshall Sir Thomas Blamey. The Naval and Military, which lasted 127 years, went into voluntary liquidation in 2009.

Sometimes, after he had spent a solid Saturday evening at one of these clubs, Beaney would recompense his wife with a Sunday morning walk on "The Block", further down Collins Street in the city centre proper. On a sunny Sunday morning, the Block was the place to see and be seen, either on the street or chatting over coffee in Gunsler's Vienna Café. An overseas observer might gaze in wonder at the variety of fashion, the colour and the conversation in this amazing city, barely 40 years old and situated at the "far end of the world" (a gentler expression than one used over a century later by the comedian Jerry Seinfeld, referring to Melbourne and by a former Australian prime minister (who shall remain nameless) referring to the country as a whole).

The Beaney social circle and activities were not confined to Collins Street, however, and, possibly driven by his longer-term political ambitions; they included amongst other events an occasional Sunday afternoon concert at the Sargoods' house in Elsternwick. Frederick Sargood, a very successful merchant, had built a fifteen-room mansion in a Lombardic style designed by Joseph Reed, the same architect who had designed the State Library and the Melbourne Town Hall. Sargood called the house Rippon Lea after his mother Emma Rippon. An elaborate and complex garden spreading over several acres surrounded the house, and orchards extended well beyond the formal garden, the whole estate covering around 45 acres. Sargood cleverly arranged to collect storm water in a large artificial lake so that the gardens and orchards were self-sufficient, even through warm summers. He kept making additions to the house over many years, adding a tower and introducing generators to supply electricity to the grand mansion and gardens.

Sargood was also a member of the Legislative Council and in his later years in Parliament assisted in the passage of some important stabilising legislation concerning stock market practices. In his earlier years however he had trouble in accommodating both his parliamentary duties and his business trips. He was assailed about this on at least one occasion and found it necessary to publicly explain (in a letter to *The Age*) a particular overseas trip as being prolonged due to a family member's illness. He wrote that he did not draw his £25 per month parliamentary stipend during his absence.

One particular evening, which was enjoyed by the doctor and Mrs. Beaney, was spent at the Mitchells'. David Mitchell, who arrived in Melbourne as a stonemason, had become very successful as a builder in his own right, his climb up the ladder at a very competitive time for builders having begun in 1856, when he successfully tendered for the masonry work on St Patrick's Cathedral in Eastern Hill. His success enabled him to acquire much property and many businesses including a brick factory, cheese and ham factories and vineyards in Coldstream and St. Hubert, just north of Melbourne. The opportunity for Mitchell and Beaney to meet occurred during the building of Scots Church, which was overseen by Mitchell, and was across the street from Beaney's house.

Early on during that particular evening Mitchell took great pride in showing his visitors the plans drawn up by the architect John Reed, for the great Exhibition building. Mitchell had won the tender to build it. Later, in addition to a violin recital by Mitchell himself, the musical entertainment included two presentations by his fourteen-year-old daughter Helen (one of ten children), whose remarkable voice and confidence were already apparent. Little did they know then of the acclaim she would receive in the great opera houses of the world, with a stage name taken from the city in which she lived.

Another enjoyable evening was an invitation to a party at Avoca, the large and beautiful South Yarra house of George and Elizabeth Kirk, with its extensive grounds running right down to the south bank of the river. It was a party to announce the engagement of their daughter Eliza to Walter Hall. Walter Hall had come from Hertfordshire to the Ballarat goldfields and was there at the time of the rebellion, but fortunately was not inside the stockade. He subsequently abandoned the pursuit of gold and became an agent for the transport firm Cobb & Co. He would later amass a fortune as a part-owner of the Mount Morgan Gold Mining Company. The particular evening of the engagement was slightly marred by a hot north wind blowing an offensive odour from a tannery across the river in Richmond. Little was said about it by anyone at the party, however, as George Kirk, who had started work in Melbourne as a butcher, owned the very large tannery. The young couple's names would later be associated with one of Australia's foremost medical research institutes, established in 1921 with a grant from them of £10,000, the Walter and Eliza Hall Institute.

When Beaney's practice allowed they might spend the weekend with the pastoralist brothers Thomas and Andrew Chirnside, at their magnificent mansion in Werribee. It consisted of fifty rooms with a unique tower, on 80 thousand acres of land, which originally had been obtained as freehold. Although neither of the Beaneys took part in sporting activities they were good conversationalists, particularly Beaney, with a glass in hand. He ensured that he remained up to date with current events, whether they were local or overseas. Some of the latter events at the time included the opening up of the Suez Canal to shorten the trip back "home", and the disappearance of the *Mary Celeste,* the American brigantine, which was found adrift in the Atlantic with her captain and crew mysteriously missing. Or conversation could be on recent publications, such as the adventures of Phileas Fogg in Jules Verne's *Around the World in 80 Days* or the new colonial novel by Marcus Clarke, *For the Term of his Natural Life,* based on convict records and legends.

A close city friend of Beaney's was James Butters, who was a share broker and gold buyer, and who was also involved in establishing the Stock Exchange in Melbourne. Beaney was godfather to his daughter Irene, who at her christening was given the middle name of Beaney; such was the strength of their friendship. A further example of that friendship was the gift of a portrait. Butters was so impressed by a portrait a little known artist by the name of Bionda had done of him (Butters) in his robes, when he was mayor of Melbourne in the late 1860s, that he commissioned the same artist to paint James Beaney in his academic robes in 1886. The portrait is now apparently in the Beaney House of Art and Knowledge – its full title – in Canterbury. Butters only had the one child, from his first wife, who had died shortly after his arrival in Melbourne from Scotland in the 1850s. He married three more times, his second wife dying in 1882 and his third wife, who was aged only 26, dying in 1885. Butters died in September 1912 at the Red Bluff Hotel in the bayside suburb of Sandringham. He was survived by his fourth wife Florence (née Forward) and the daughter, Irene Beaney Butters.

In 1890, one year before James Beaney died, he "came down" with a very severe chest infection and was advised by his physician, Dr. Williams, to stop work for a month and seek some bayside air. He spent that month at the Red Bluff Hotel. Unfortunately the Red Bluff, with its beautiful façade and extensive bay views, was bulldozed in 2005 after it had been gutted by fire.

The goings on in local politics and in the building societies was a fairly constant topic and Beaney could hold his audience without being boring. In sharp contrast to parts of his medical world he was generally a welcome guest, despite his flamboyance, or because of it, and his evident "nouveau riche" manner.

Mary Beaney, although of a much quieter disposition, particularly in her husband's presence, was exceedingly knowledgeable in horticultural matters and welcomed the opportunity to view the indigenous flora, which contrasted so strongly with her more familiar English and Welsh countryside. She had already, along with a small band of like-minded colonials, written to the *Argus* expressing concern about the wholesale felling of trees in the colony, especially the red gums. She was mindful however not to press her views too strongly in the presence of her hosts, even though there was evidence around her of aggressive clearing. At Werribee few trees had been spared except for the river area where the tall gums, providing cool and shady banks on the Werribee River, remained secure. It was also of regret to her that their own opulent house, so convenient for her husband's hospital and private practice, denied her the pleasure of a larger garden. She most likely had mixed feelings when, that year on Empire Day, the Mayor of Melbourne, James Gatehouse, an eccentric hat importer and maker, planted the first trees in Collins Street, as they were not natives.

Another convenience of the location of their Collins Street house, not admitted openly by Beaney, was its nearness to Bear and Ford's depot (at 83 Little Collins St) which handled his favourite Victorian wines from Tabilk. The Tabilk vineyard, which was established at Nagambie in the Goulburn Valley in 1860, produced a good quality wine, which would later win the

Diploma of Honour, the highest award given, at the greater London Exhibition in 1899. It was Tabilk wine that Beaney always insisted be taken on board the Golden Crown on their annual summer trip to Sorrento, at the south end of Port Phillip Bay. Many relaxing holiday evenings were spent at Sorrento, either partying near Coppin's amphitheatre or engaging in lengthy conversation with such fellow holiday makers as Edmond Finn who later, writing as 'Garryowen', would chronicle much of Melbourne's early history. Another fellow holidaymaker on the peninsula was the up and coming young lawyer Frank Gavan Duffy. Following his admission to the Bar four years passed before he obtained a brief, but his skills rapidly became evident and subsequently he often appeared with or against James Purves, the two being regarded as the best trial lawyers of the time. Incidentally Gavan Duffy was himself involved in the crash following the land boom and paid his creditors only 3d. (3 pence) in the pound at the time and obtained a clear discharge. Years later he apparently paid out his debts in full.

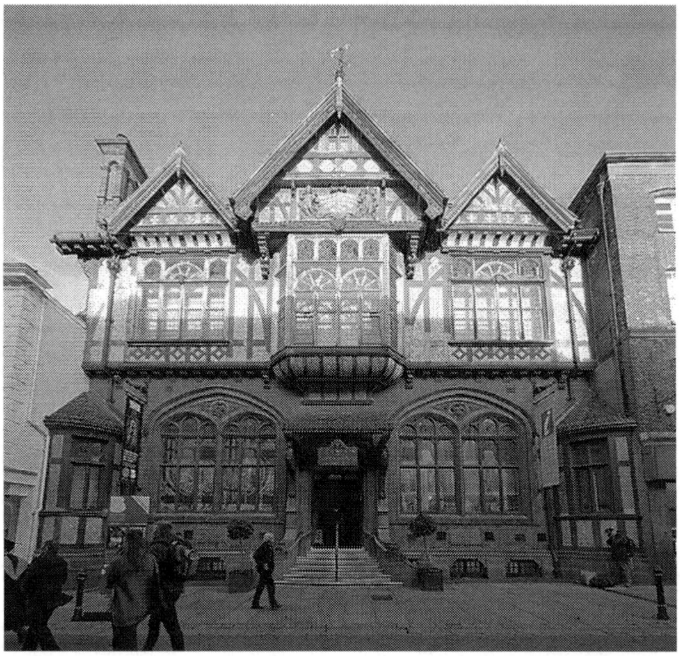

Figure 9: Beaney House of Art and Knowledge, Canterbury, UK.

Beaney's private practice was also, to an extent, a reflection of his social success with many of his patients being from the moneyed (new) and/or political world. Sometimes it was difficult to separate the work from the pleasure. For example, a consultation at Osborne House, up on Nicholson Street in Fitzroy, to attend to the ex-Premier John McPherson, would end up with a pleasant drink in the forecourt and a discussion on the political issues of the day. McPherson had been Premier in the period 1869-70, a very volatile time in Victorian politics. Or towards evening Beaney might call on Thomas Ewing, a Fitzroy pharmacist, for supplies of medicine but spend an hour sampling his quinine wine, amongst other liquids. It was the bitter taste of quinine in tonic water that made the mix of gin and tonic so popular with British colonials in India in the late 1800s.

Much was going on, or rather not going on depending upon one's political views, in the Victorian Parliament at that time. George Kerford, who had been Premier for less than twelve months, surprisingly resigned when the Parliament divided over his bill to increase taxes. He could have weathered the event, as he still had a majority of one, but he recognised how unpopular the bill was.

As soon as his successor, Graham Berry, was installed by the acting Governor Sir William Stawell in August 1875, he introduced a bill for the establishment of protective tariffs. Berry wished to protect the rapidly growing manufacturing interests in Melbourne from the much cheaper Asian imports, particularly of furniture, clothing, hats and footwear. Despite his gift of fiery oratory, however, he could not get his bill through. He asked Stawell to dissolve the house. Stawell, a former judge and a very diligent and conscientious administrator, refused to do so, his sympathies lying with the conservatives rather than with Berry and the democrats. The Victorian town of Stawell (of the Stawell Gift) is appropriately named after him, as the well-built and tall Stawell was an excellent sportsman. Instead of dissolving the House, Stawell summoned James McCulloch to form a new Administration. It was the 17th government in as many years. McCulloch led against Barry's Opposition group from November but not much was achieved until March 1876 as the Opposition stonewalled, to delay the conduct of any business. The papers of the day reported that the Government was gagged by an 'iron hand', in an almost farcical situation.

It is doubtful if the appointed Governor, Sir George Bowen, who was absent overseas during 1875, could have done much more than Stawell to improve the situation if he had been present. Sir George was a well-educated man, having gained an Oxford "first" in classics, but was quite egocentric. He loved to quote Latin and Greek (rarely giving a translation) and enjoyed the pomp and ceremony of his post.

He opened many railway lines during his term, travelling in style in a special carriage, unlike a previous Governor, Latrobe, who would turn up alone and on horseback, to perform his duties. One of Bowen's favourite quotes was 'We English are the true "gens togata"' (those entitled to wear the Roman toga). On his way "home", on that year of leave, he stopped in Italy and met with King Victor Emmanuel, Pope Pius IX and Giuseppe Garibaldi. He conversed with them all in Italian but, being aware of the loyalty fluctuations in Italian politics, he did not tell each one he was seeing the other. On his way back to Australia he visited the Governor General in Canada and President Ulysses S. Grant in America. His visit with the latter was very brief, probably because at that time President Grant had significant problems to address in the South with outlaws, some of whom were ex-Confederate soldiers, and in the west with native American tribes, resentful of being deprived of their land and their way of life.

On his return to Victoria in January 1876 Bowen and his Italian wife Diamentina, the daughter of Count Condiano Di Roma, stayed at Bishopcourt in Clarendon Street, East Melbourne, until the new Government House was completed in mid year. Once ensconced in her new surroundings Lady Diamentina began her series of "small and earlys", as they came to be called. These were weekly parties for 30 to 40 people with singing, dancing and light refreshments in the State dining room. Being also versed in the classical languages the Collins Street doctors (and lawyers), with their partners, were not infrequent guests at these functions so it is likely that the Beaneys were invited, but there is no record of their having attended.

One political point, for which Governor Bowen is justifiably recalled, was his speaking out on the shameful ministerial patronage that was associated with senior appointments to the public service. However that was probably the extent of his entry into the intrigue and understanding of colonial politics. Even if he had arrived back in Melbourne in time, it is also unlikely that he would or could have intervened to assist Beaney in avoiding the further public embarrassment, which was to involve this prominent surgeon.

5. Two problem cases and the consequences

Towards the end of 1875 Beaney operated upon two male patients, each resulting in a tragic outcome. The first was Michael Barrie, a fifteen-year-old boy with a crippling problem of a painful, deformed and stiff hip, possibly due to a past infection, although the cause was never established.

In the operation, which Beaney claimed was his own unique procedure, he attempted to create a false joint by dividing the neck of the femur (the long thigh bone) below the hip joint. He expected that the hip and thigh muscles would allow the limb to move freely but retain sufficient control and stability for him to weight bear and to walk, albeit with a shortened leg. The operation was performed under chloroform anaesthesia, administered by a Dr. Lewellin. The procedure was almost finished when the boy stopped breathing and several minutes later his heart stopped.

Reports of the efforts to revive him, as became clear in the subsequent Coroner's inquest, were conflicting. The inquest had been held because the case was one of "death on the table", under chloroform. Such events, with chloroform, would concern the medical profession and the public for at least another fifty years.

The second patient was actually admitted to the hospital in November but not operated upon until early December. This case, which became more of a cause célèbre involved a relatively young man, Robert Berth, who had been sent from Amherst Hospital, in the mid-Victorian goldfields region, to Dr. John Webb, in his capacity as an assistant surgeon at the Melbourne Hospital.

Berth was suffering from a stone in the bladder. He was very weak and had been an inmate of Amherst Hospital for some considerable time before being referred to the Melbourne Hospital. The stone was believed to be large and the doctors at Amherst requested that he be operated upon as soon as possible. Webb, having privileges to attend to outpatients only, referred him to Dr. Beaney. On the 30th November, several days after the patient's admission, Dr. Beaney examined him in the presence of his house surgeon and medical students. He found the patient to be thin, pale and haggard with a rapid and weak pulse. Beaney introduced a sound (a long metal probe) into the patient's bladder and found it to be thickened and contracted around a large stone. The procedure caused much discomfort and Beaney did not persist for long. He ordered that the patient have as much nourishment as he could take and planned to operate on December 2nd. He also ordered that the patient's bowels be well cleared out by an enema before the operation was undertaken.

In the operating room on December 2nd, as the patient was being placed on the table, Beaney clarified that the bowels had been emptied and received confirmation from the house surgeon that they had indeed been well cleared out. The same resident physician, Dr. Lewellin, administered a chloroform anaesthetic and Berth was placed in the lithotomy position (on his back with his legs spread apart and each held elevated in stirrups), to display the lower part of the buttocks and the perineum, which is that part of the body between the scrotum and the anus.

With a sizeable audience, Beaney, in his favourite and none too clean white coat, buttoned up to protect his vest, but with diamonds and rubies still adorning his otherwise bare hands, seated himself in front of the patient's buttocks. He plunged a scalpel into the skin in the midline in front of the anus, cut upwards then backwards on to a silver speculum, which had been placed in the rectum, thus cutting through the anterior wall of the rectum, but not its posterior wall, which was protected by the speculum.

He continued to cut upwards through the prostate gland, which sits below the bladder, and then passed a long silver director up through the same incision and into the bladder. He introduced his right index finger along the track so made and widened it to allow the finger to enter the bladder. He passed a stone forceps along his finger up into the bladder and seized the stone but found it to be larger than was first suspected. The forceps kept slipping off the stone.

With the stone now being visible at the orifice of the wound many attempts were made to remove it, with the invariable result of the stone slipping off the forceps and the removal of only small fragments.

With sweat beginning to appear on his forehead, an event unusual for Beaney, and amid murmuring amongst the audience, Beaney contemplated his options. He decided against an approach from the front, that is the abdominal or suprapubic approach, as this required the bladder to be distended to avoid injuring the bowel, a mishap, which he knew was likely to result in peritonitis and death. He knew also that the bladder he was dealing with here would not expand due to its chronically infected and contracted condition. An alternative was to crush the stone, but the ordinary lithotrities (instruments used to crush bladder stones) in the Melbourne Hospital were not large enough or strong enough to accomplish this.

After some contemplation he obtained two metal lithotomy scoops and passed one up behind and one in front of the stone and with his assistant, Dr. Webb, dragging on one scoop and he on the other, the stone was drawn down and eventually fell to the floor. It was rather irregular in shape but appeared to the audience to be about three inches (over seven cm) in diameter. Its weight subsequently was found to be six and a half ounces (nearly 200 gm).

A large catheter was introduced into the bladder, which was then washed out with warm water, the water freely flowing back through the surgical wound which Beaney had made in the perineum. The patient was then returned to the ward with orders to receive morphine for pain relief and to be given beef tea at regular intervals, with as much champagne as he could drink.

Beaney visited the patient early on the following morning and found him to be well, with urine flowing freely from the bladder through the perineal wound. Although his pulse was rapid his temperature was normal, he had not vomited and he had no tenderness in the abdomen. He was less well however on December 5th, when Beaney again visited him. His pulse was now even more rapid and feeble, he had been vomiting and he was markedly "drawn" in appearance. His voice had gone to a whisper and there was tenderness all over the abdomen. He complained of pain in his back and of coldness in his limbs. He was putting out very little urine. When Beaney asked him what he would like, his faint reply was port wine. He gradually became weaker and died shortly before midnight. Beaney considered the cause of death as acute pyelitis or "surgical kidney".

Some days later, whether it was through his enormous vanity and egotism, as his critics would claim, or his wish to share with the world his fascination with the medical curiosity of such a large stone, Beaney had a facsimile of it made. This was then mounted and displayed together with a smaller stone, one and a half ounces in weight, which had been removed from another patient twelve months beforehand, in the window of a Collins Street bookshop near his home.

As he had been re-elected there was no immediate need to advertise but there may have been another practical reason for the display, and that was to advertise his textbooks. These were on sale in the same shop, which was owned by Ferdinand Baillière. Beaney had written nothing since 1873 and his book sales may have needed a boost. His output of publications had been constant and plentiful up until that year, but criticism was about that he had at times plagiarised some authors' works and that, at other times, a ghost writer was engaged by him, or by Baillière, to produce a paper for an important address. Such an address or lecture would subsequently be published unashamedly with Beaney as the sole author. Clearly there was an awareness in the medical community of possible plagiarism as an unnamed author wrote, in the *Medical Gazette,* that 'Nobody accuses Mr. Beaney of being able to write ten consecutive lines of readable English'.

Melbourne's weather then, as now, was notorious for sudden and often unseasonable changes. It was wet and cold in the two weeks before Christmas 1875, and Melburnians had plenty of time to read an editorial and a spate of letters, relating to Beaney's practice, which appeared in a morning paper over the next ten days.

The *Argus,* which was published in Melbourne up until 1957, was the paper involved. The second leading article of its issue on Friday December 17th reported the findings of the inquest on the death of the boy Barrie, following the hip operation.

It was a very aggressive leader, indicating that Dr. Beaney had broken Rule 7 of the hospital, concerning the necessity for consultations with colleagues prior to an important operation, that he was "too clever by half", and that his rushing the boy to operation was reprehensible and cruel in the extreme. It concluded that Beaney's conduct was highly censurable and that he should cut down on his surgery as soon as possible.

Predictably, Beaney was furious. He immediately wrote a letter to the editor, had it delivered that morning, and it was published the very next day. In that letter Beaney defended his decision to operate and went on to claim that the operation he had performed was one he had personally developed for such a condition, as most others had been unsuccessful. Perhaps if he had not written that letter, with his provocative claim for originality with this particular operation, subsequent events may have been different.

Also in the *Argus* on that Saturday, December 18th, along with Beaney's response, was a letter to the editor from Dr. Alex Fisher, a Collins Street surgeon, supportive of Dr. Beaney. It posed a question mark as to Dr. Lewellin's skills and actions, suggesting that

Lewellin had been more interested in the operation than the anaesthetic he was administering, and had demonstrated an inappropriate delay in resuscitation of the patient.

Obviously much discussion and much ink were expended over that weekend for there were five letters in the Monday December 20th edition of the *Argus.*

Under the heading 'Death under chloroform' there was a letter from Dr. Lewellin asking the public to wait upon any comments about the performance of the anaesthetic until the results of a review, being conducted on the issue by the hospital, were available. There were two separate letters of support for Dr. Lewellin, one from a surgeon, Dr. A. Wilkins and one from a person signing as EBH. Concerning this second letter of support there may have been a misreading of the hand written 'E' (by the typesetter) and the correspondent may well have been George Britton Halford, the respected professor of anatomy.

Beaney would have read all of the above letters with interest and concern but his interest and concern must have turned to distress as he read the fifth letter in the *Argus* that morning. It was a long letter, dated December 18th, and was simply signed 'A Practical Surgeon'.

In the first part there was a response to Beaney's letter, which had appeared on the Saturday, about the "so called" Beaney operation and stated that the operation that Beaney claimed to be new was not so, but had been performed by Dr. Barton of Philadelphia in 1826, with success. The Practical Surgeon went on to say that if James Beaney was so keen to have his operations brought to the public notice, there were two others, which he performed at the Melbourne Hospital less than three weeks before, without consultation with his colleagues.

One was excision of a knee joint, in which the intention had been to excise a diseased joint and bring the long bones together to arthrodese or stiffen the joint. The cutting had been done poorly, so the letter claimed, and the bones would not fit. Amputation was then resorted to and this was performed at too low a level, in fact it was performed through the problem area of bone.

The second case referred to by A Practical Surgeon was the operation on a man with a bladder stone (the operation detailed above on Robert Berth). The letter continued:

> The second or lithotomy case was put upon the table. The patient was a young and healthy man. Mr. Beaney stated to the students that as the stone was small he would perform the median operation; however, he attempted the trans-rectal or Lloyd's method. After some considerable cutting he got into the bladder, but only to find that the stone was an unusually large one.

Having failed, after strenuous efforts, to remove it, a bystander requested him to crush the stone. This advice, however, he would not take, as he stated he was most anxious to extract it whole. There were two other operations still open to him to save the patient's life, viz, the bilateral, or the suprapubic. He did not avail himself of either, but continued pulling and pulling and bending the hospital instruments, endeavouring to extract the large stone through the small opening. By sheer force the much – prized lump was hauled out. The result of course is easy to imagine – the man died of peritonitis.

Now, Sir, had Mr. Beaney taken the advice tendered to him, and crushed the stone, it is almost a certainty that the man would now be alive. A cast of the stone is on view at a bookseller's in Collins Street East as an advertisement for Mr. Beaney's great operative skill, but the poor man from whom this great specimen was extracted is in his grave. I wonder what reason Mr. Beaney will give the committee for not calling a consultation on these two cases. Perhaps they are exclusively his own operations, and that he feared his colleagues not understanding them might veto his chance of displaying such an amount of surgical skill.

– I am, & c., Dec 18. A Practical Surgeon.

Beaney felt that he had been maligned by a deceitful staff member. To him the letter was filled with exaggeration and sarcasm. He did not know exactly who the writer was, or where the writer got the idea that Berth had died with peritonitis, but quite reasonably presumed it was one of the other surgeons connected with the Melbourne Hospital.

That morning the newly appointed Minister for Justice, Mr. John Madden, also read the letters in the *Argus.* He was young for the position and keen to be seen as being on top of his role. Certain parts of the letter aroused his concern: 'Two other operations still open to him to save the patient's life, he did not avail himself of either, ''by sheer force', and lastly, 'the man died of peritonitis'. He also put a question mark beside the words 'a cast of the stone is on view at a bookseller's in Collins Street'. Later, in his office that morning, the Minister for Justice summoned Police Inspector Green and his Departmental secretary to a conference about the implications of the letter. On the face of it the letter suggested willful and criminal negligence on the part of Dr. Beaney.

Because of Beaney's prominence, both medically and socially, it was determined in the first instance that two senior detectives, Duncan and Gould, should make discreet enquires amongst the resident doctors at the Melbourne Hospital and report back to him within three days. The Minister did not want the issue hanging over through the forthcoming holiday period.

Meanwhile Beaney, calmed down somewhat by his wife and a medicinal brandy (or two) sent a note to his friend and solicitor Joe Duffett, requesting Duffett to join him for lunch at his Club. Duffett had established a very successful law practice and was a well-known figure in Melbourne as a decade before he had been requested to handle the issue of the nineteen American sailors, who had deserted the *CSS Shenandoah,* the Confederate ship that had sought sanctuary and repairs in Melbourne towards the end of the American Civil War. When the ship left Melbourne no one knew about the forty-two Australians who had been secretly (and illegally) taken on board as crew, the ship being chronically undermanned because of the Confederate Force's chronic shortage of funds.

Hurrying through his consultations that morning, Beaney was in no mood for patient chitchat. Fortunately most of their complaints seemed minor, compared with the problem with which he was grappling.

When they met, Beaney quickly told Buffett of the "stone case", its outcome and the contents of the letter. He pointed out the phrases which he considered to be deceitful: 'a young and healthy patient', 'two other operations to save his life'; the exaggerations 'by sheer force' and 'hauled out'. He also highlighted what he considered sarcasm: 'the much prized stone' and 'Beaney's great skill'; and finally the writer's presumption concerning the cause of death 'died of peritonitis'.

Beaney ran through a longer list of surgeons than just his three senior colleagues. Could it be Fitzgerald, James, Howett, Barker or Webb? He felt that the last named was the least likely, being his junior and having being part of the operating team. He felt that Barker was the most likely, having still not got over his defeat at the recent elections.

Beaney was keen to press for an action against the writer of the letter but Duffett indicated the obvious, namely that he could not sue an unknown writer. He promised however, that as he had a passing acquaintance with the editor of the *Argus,* he would make appropriate enquires. He well knew that the editor, as with the priest and confessor, would not divulge his source, but his offer had the intended calming effect on Beaney, who then settled down to his champagne and luncheon, vowing never to buy the *Argus* again. Like the fate of many resolutions, however, this vow lasted only a day or two. Besides who knew what next dastardly attack might be made on its pages in a further effort to "bring him down."

Conscious of the Minister's words about the need for discretion in this case, Detectives Duncan and Gould interviewed the resident surgeon, George Annand and the resident physician, John Williams, who were both present at the operation. They also interviewed James Duncan (no relation), who was not present at the operation, but who purported to know all about the hospital's instruments. They were interviewed separately in the morning and then together in the afternoon, during which meeting sketches were made of the operation performed, as well as some alternative operations which were available to Beaney. They told the detectives of their knowledge of the patient, the operation and of the various instruments used. The detectives were a little surprised at the frankness in their description of the procedure with words such as 'great force being used', 'persisting for an unusually long time', etc.

The residents could not however agree upon the cause of death. Perhaps it was from peritonitis. They did not know, but they were fairly sure it was the operation and nothing to do with the after-care provided by the resident staff. Perhaps, unknown to the detectives, they had determined that it was better to be offside with one surgeon than with the other three, whom they knew to be of one mind about Beaney. To the resident staff Beaney was a rather eccentric person. Admittedly he was quite a character and the hospital, being a dismal place at times certainly needed characters, but he also could be unreasonably sharp. They had all experienced more than one dressing down for not having followed his instructions exactly. They had occasionally also to accept the blame for a poor outcome, which they believed was influenced more by the consultant than any lack of attention and skill on their part. However such experiences occurred with the other surgeons as well.

The next day, having summarised the resident doctors' reports, Detective Duncan interviewed Dr. John Webb at his house in East Melbourne. Duncan showed Webb his summary and asked him if he agreed with its contents. Webb did agree. Duncan then obtained Webb's own opinion of the operation, of the manner in which it had been carried out and in particular what other options were available to Dr. Beaney. Webb spoke fairly quickly and Duncan, perhaps unwisely, made only occasional notes, finalising his report back at the Department late on the evening of December 22nd.

The police report of their enquiries was sent to the Coroner, Dr. Youl, on the morning of December 23rd. On reviewing the report Dr. Youl then ordered that the body of Robert Berth be exhumed, that a post-mortem be conducted on the body and that an inquest on the circumstances of his death be held on Wednesday December 29th. He issued a summons to Dr. Beaney to attend. Being informed of the Coroner's decisions the Minister acquiesced. Indeed having instigated the inquiry he could do little else, but he advised Dr. Youl that the Crown would not provide a prosecutor and that he, the Coroner, should ensure that the case for the Crown was appropriately presented and heard. The Minister, himself a barrister, further advised that in the interests of justice Mr. Beaney could have legal representation.

On December 24th whilst the body was being exhumed the Coroner endeavoured to obtain unprejudiced persons to perform the post-mortem examination. He applied to Professor Halford, Professor of Anatomy at the University, who refused. It may be that Professor Halford appreciated Beaney's support and interest in student teaching and was well disposed towards him. Halford had, incidentally, been called in as a supporting witness for Beaney in the 1860s "abortion" case to re-examine the deceased. Or it may simply have been because it was required to be done on Christmas Day.

Dr. Lawrence, the Demonstrator of Anatomy, had already gone on holiday and was unavailable. His third choice, Dr. Rudall, the pathologist at the Melbourne Hospital, also declined to conduct the post-mortem. Mr. Barker, the Lecturer in Surgery at the University, (the same man who had until recently been a member of the honorary surgical staff at the Melbourne Hospital) agreed to undertake the duty. Dr. Neild, the Lecturer on Medical Jurisprudence at the University, and a member of the medical staff at the hospital, also agreed to do so.

It was known that Dr. Youl himself was not enamoured of the Melbourne Hospital. So many of the cases, which had passed before him, were deaths related to infection, which he believed was due to the hospital environment. Some years later, when these views were made public, he received much criticism for his perceived biases.

Being the eve of Christmas, Beaney had already planned to have only a few consultations that day and spent some hours again with Duffett in the afternoon discussing how they should proceed. They had both agreed that a barrister should be instructed and Duffett, that morning, had been to various barristers' chambers to engage one. He told Dr. Beaney that unfortunately most of the senior men with whom he had worked, and whose skills he respected, were either already away, or intended to be away in the following week. He had however, been fortunate in obtaining the services of a young up and coming barrister of whom he had heard excellent reports. He withheld from Beaney comments that one or two of his colleagues had made that this young barrister's youthful aggression could sometimes put judges a little off side. The barrister's name was James Liddell Purves. Dr. Beaney accepted Duffett's recommendation and a note was sent to Mr. Purves asking him to meet them the morning after Christmas Day at Beaney's house in Collins Street.

The post-mortem was conducted at the morgue on Christmas morning, by Drs. Barker and Neild, with Dr. Beaney, Dr. Fisher and several other medical men in attendance.

The following account is from the official report made for the hospital by Dr. Alex Fisher, with some minor technical points (in the conduct of the autopsy) omitted.

NOTES OF THE *Post-mortem* APPEARANCES OF THE BODY OF ROBERT BERTH, ON WHOM THE OPERATION OF LITHOTOMY HAD BEEN PERFORMED BY MR BEANEY AT THE MELBOURNE HOSPITAL.

Saturday, December 25th, 11.45a.m.

The body was found to be in an advanced state of decomposition, and covered by maggots, and had to be well washed with the hose before being subjected to examination. The features were swollen and unrecognisable. The skin, on the trunk and limbs, was of a pale greenish colour, and the epidermis of the whole body peeled off, even from the soles of the feet. The penis was much swollen, and the scrotum distended with gas.

There was a wound in the perineum 3 1/2 inches long, and about 1 1/4 inches broad in its widest part; its edges were everted and decomposed. The body having been placed in the lithotomy position, the external wound was examined and found to communicate with the rectum by passing a probe from above downwards. The head having being opened, the brain was found in a semi fluid state, and could not be examined. The heart and lungs were much decomposed, no apparent disease being present. On opening the abdomen, no effusion of serum or blood was found in its cavity. The liver appeared of normal size, and was of a dark dirty-green colour, and much decomposed. The intestines were in tolerably good preservation, and were of a pale colour, and presented no appearance of inflammation or of effused lymph. On turning over the bowels the large intestine was found attached to the external wall of the abdomen by old and firm adhesions. The stomach and intestines were opened, and found to be healthy. The small intestine contained excrement the colour of yellow ochre and the descending colon and rectum were filled with dark solid faeces. Several parts of the small intestine and mesentery were removed by Dr. Barker and placed in a jar with spirits and water. The spleen and pancreas appeared to be healthy. The kidneys and the ureters were dissected from their attachments. Some decomposed blood which had accumulated in the pelvis during this procedure was removed and placed in a separate bottle. There was no appearance of infiltration of urine, or of inflammation of the cellular structures of the pelvis. The pelvis was divided on each side of the pubis and the bladder and rectum removed. On examining the kidneys, the left was found inflamed, but otherwise healthy; the lining membrane of the ureter of the same side was of a pale colour throughout until about within three inches of the bladder. The right kidney was larger than its fellow, and was of a deep purple colour throughout its whole structure, which was softened. It contained in its substance two calculi, one of considerable size and of irregular shape.

> The lining membrane of the right ureter was also of a dark red colour throughout its whole extent. The bladder on being opened was found to be very much thickened. Its mucous membrane, being of a dark port wine colour throughout, had its whole surface covered with a phosphatic deposit, which was firmly adherent. The prostate gland was dilated almost to an extent beyond recognition. The rectum was lacerated to the extent of one and a-half inches from its orifice through the muscular coats, and for about half an inch further through the mucous membrane only.
>
> (Signed) ALEXANDER FISHER, L.R.C.S., Edin.

On the Sunday morning (Boxing Day) Duffett introduced the barrister, James Purves, to James Beaney. He must have noted that the only thing they had in common was their first name. His surgical friend, in middle age with rounded cheeks and ample girth, clothed in one of his usual colourful weskits and his bejewelled watch and chain, contrasted strongly with his young legal colleague's sharp features, slight build and sombre attire. Nor of course did the contrast escape the astute Mr. Purves, who decided, within a few minutes, that Beaney's garish appearance and his self-assertive bearing would not win sympathy from a jury. He would not call Beaney in front of the jury to give evidence.

Purves, however, also noted Beaney's extensive library, covering two walls of his consulting room, and before they sat down Purves moved from cabinet to cabinet, quickly eyeing the various medical texts and journals on display. Over what to Purves was an unnecessarily elaborate morning coffee, prepared by Mary Beaney for the three men and brought in by their East Indian servant, the details and problem issues of the case, and the situation in which Beaney was placed, were discussed. At the conclusion of the conference Purves told Beaney that he would most likely not call him to give evidence.

This news was disconcerting to Beaney, but Duffett advised that he was now in the barrister's hands and he must allow Purves to act as he saw fit. In the brief time they had been meeting Duffett had recognised his young colleague's sharp intellect and also his determination.

These qualities were in later years to make Purves the most prominent of advocates, with an involvement in the majority of major court cases in the city for over thirty years and he was regarded as being amongst the State's great advocates. One of the longest and most publicised cases concerned his defence of David Syme the proprietor of *The Age,* which had published a series of articles highly critical of Richard Speight, the Railways Commissioner, who it claimed was under the influence of a number of members of Parliament, members who were in effect developers, and who were profiting from the various railway extensions through land they themselves had purchased. The *Argus,* hoping to damage Syme, the editor and part owner of their main rival (*The Age*), supported Speight. Defending Speight was Gavan Duffy, who by then was as well regarded in his profession, as was Purves. The court case took nine months, with the initial verdict decided against Syme, but the appeal case that followed took a further five months, with Purves ultimately achieving a victory for Syme.

James Purves was born in Melbourne but educated in Europe, being sent there at the age of 12, as his health was poor, quite the opposite of Beaney who was sent away from the cold northern climate because of his poor health. He was admitted to the Bar in 1865. He was to become known also as a sportsman and politician and would move in high social and political circles. He joined the Australian Natives' Association (ANA) in 1872 and was its President in the years 1888-90. Despite the title the ANA had nothing to do with indigenous activities. It was a mutual society founded in Melbourne in 1871 and membership was restricted to Australian-born men, mainly of Anglo-Saxon origin. It was extended to the other Australian colonies in 1872. As well as a social benefit it provided sickness, medical and funeral insurance cover and membership was sought after by young men keen to make their way in the country. During his tenure as President his forthright and firm manner led to Purves being referred to as the

"Emperor". The impressive list of members, with whom Purves would have mixed at that time included Edmond Barton, Australia's first Prime Minister, Alfred Deakin, who succeeded Barton when he went to the High Court, Isaac Isaacs, Australia's first Australian-born Governor General and Henry Parkes, the Father of Federation. Alfred Deakin was also a barrister and continued to work as such for a number of years after he had entered Parliament. One case Deakin was involved in received a great deal of publicity both in Victoria and overseas. He unsuccessfully defended a notorious villain called Frederick Deeming, who was charged with murdering his wife, Emily, in the Melbourne suburb of Windsor in 1891. It subsequently transpired that at the time of his marriage to Emily he was a bigamist, with a wife and four children in Rainhill, England. Tragically it was discovered that he had murdered the first wife and all of the children, just a matter of months after his second marriage took place. Because of the manner of the deaths, either by strangling or cutting the victims' throats, the newspapers in London and New York raised the question of Deeming possibly being the notorious Jack the Ripper, as he was in London in 1888 at the time of the equally savage Whitechapel murders.

The ANA reduced its political activity after Federation was achieved in 1901, but continued to prosper as a health fund, building society, insurer and fund manager until 1993, when it merged with the Manchester Unity to become Australian Unity.

In keeping with his prosperity, Charles Webb would design Purves's future mansion, Mosspennock, in East Melbourne. Webb was the architect for many other fine buildings including Melbourne Grammar School, the Windsor Hotel, Tasma Terrace and the Alfred Hospital. Mosspennock, which is still standing, as are the other buildings mentioned, was erected next door to Cliveden, Sir William Clarke's magnificent town house, which had around thirty bedrooms. Clarke's house was located on the corner of Clarendon Street and Wellington Parade. It is now the site of a large hotel, which was the Hilton and is now called Pullman Melbourne on the Park, and Mosspennock is the large and handsome white building directly behind it in Clarendon Street. Mosspennock is in the process of being converted to luxury units.

Sir William Clarke was the son of an unremarkable Tasmanian butcher. When he came over to Victoria in 1837 he bought up a large amount of land in the colony at just one pound an acre. The other great mansion Clarke had built was Ruperstwood in Sunbury where he and his wife, Janet (née Snodgrass) entertained on a grand scale. It was there, in 1882, that Janet, Lady Clarke, presented a small urn of ashes (probably of a bail) to Mr. Ivo Bligh, the captain of the touring English cricket team, during a game between the Australian cricketers and the "gentlemen" members of the touring team, played at Rupertswood.

Mr. Bligh returned to Australia in 1884 and married Lady Clarke's music teacher, Florence Murphy. They lived in Powlett Street, East Melbourne for some years, close to the Clarkes, but on the death of his brother in England Bligh became the Earl of Darnley and inherited Cobham Hall, a Tudor era mansion in Kent, which is now an independent day and boarding school for girls.

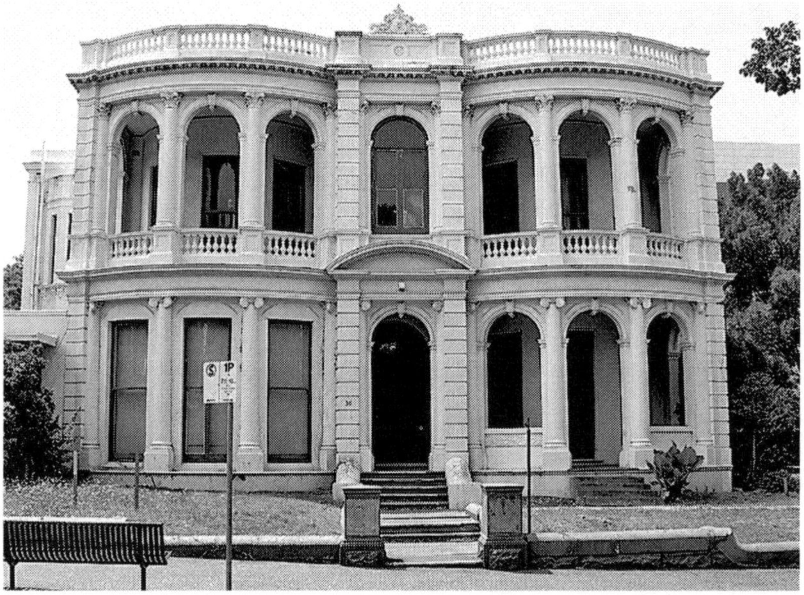

Figure 10: Mosspennoch mansion, East Melbourne.

When the Earl died, the urn was given by Lady Darnley (née Murphy) to the Marylebone Cricket Club. It remains today in the Long Room at the Lord's Pavilion (cricket ground) and of course is the basis for the prized Ashes cricket contest of Test matches regularly played, and keenly fought, between England and Australia. Sir William Clarke was made an hereditary baronet by Queen Victoria for having been

President of the successful 1880-1881 Melbourne Exhibition.

His courtroom wit would occasionally lead Purves to a "fall". A very public and literal one occurred many years later when, in response to an insult by Purves in court, a Dr H.M. O'Hara accosted him in Collins Street and knocked him into the gutter. Purves had, during a cross-examination of the doctor, queried a large fee of £1000 charged by O'Hara, asking facetiously 'Was it for a legal or illegal operation?' The pugilistic incident made the daily papers. It was a pity they could not have hit it off in a more cordial way by recognising their mutual interest in horse racing. O'Hara had a horse called Ben Bolt, which won a Caulfield Cup and Purves, whose father was a horse breeder, was said to have owned a number of fine racehorses. Horses of course in that period held the interest of the people in the way that the motorcar does today. Even the surgeon Thomas Fitzgerald had a number of horses, and won the Victorian Grand National Hurdle in 1882, with a horse called Rhesus. Only the occasional professional man today has such an interest in horse racing, although it might be stronger in the legal than the medical profession.

Dr. O'Hara was an honorary surgeon at the Alfred Hospital at the time of the confrontation and was also in private practice in Collins Street, where he had in 1892 purchased the late James Beaney's large Cromwell House. O'Hara added to the house by building a private hospital on its Russell Street side.

O'Hara was regarded as a good surgeon and a good teacher although he was sometimes contradictory and inconsistent in his statements. He had an excellent speaking voice and was also a gifted baritone, often singing in public and was at one time encouraged by Dame Nellie Melba to take up a career as a singer. He was tall and solidly built and usually of a genial disposition but his Irish (Cork) temper could be stirred at times. Whereas Purves had initially commenced a medical course and switched to law, O'Hara commenced studying law at Melbourne University in 1872, but found it uncongenial and went back to Ireland and transferred to medicine, graduating in Dublin. Perceiving no other means of redress and smoldering over the issue for days he took the rather unprofessional and more direct approach mentioned above, when he chanced upon Purves in the street. Unfortunately Purves's sporting powers had not extended to boxing, and as his aggressive court manner was by then well known, he did not get much public sympathy.

The sporting interests of James Purves did include tennis and yachting. He once had the loan of Sir William Clarke's yacht *The Janet,* during Sir William's absence overseas in 1890, but his major interest clearly was in purchasing and breeding fine racehorses. Early in 1875 he had married Lavinia, daughter of Richard Grice, a member of the Committee of Management of the Melbourne Hospital. Tragically

Lavinia was later to die in childbirth, having previously delivered a healthy son.

In 1879 Purves was married again, this time to Eliza Emma Broadribb and they subsequently had five children. Eliza's father, William Adams Broadribb, owned an enormous run of nearly 450 square miles of land, on the Lachlan and Murrumbidgee rivers in New South Wales, and his brothers owned another 250 square miles. At the time of the forthcoming inquest in 1875, however, there was just Purves and his new young wife, Lavinia, and he was keenly building up his legal practice.

Purves quickly followed his decision not to have him as a witness with a request that Beaney set out for him the full details of his acquaintance with Robert Berth. He also asked for information on Beaney's own preparation for the operation, his orders for the preparation of the patient, the details of the operation itself, the subsequent care and terminal events, and also the details of the postmortem. Beaney agreed to do so.

Purves also indicated the constraints under which he would be working. These included his limited knowledge of surgery and the stone operation in particular, and the difficulty he would have in obtaining access to the necessary medical information, as all libraries would be closed over the holiday period (how fortunate we are with the internet). He motioned to Beaney's books and ventured that his difficulties would be reduced if Beaney could draw from his grand library the related texts, and index for him relevant passages from recognised authorities. He pointed out that this was the most practical way for Beaney to assist with his defence. Recognising the opportunity this provided him to impart the right information to Purves, Beaney agreed to do so.

Purves requested permission to spend the following day there in Beaney's consulting rooms digesting the necessary information. He further said that he wished to be able to work without interruption and suggested that Beaney should find some distraction from the forthcoming events.

The improvement in the weather, which was certainly warmer than the previous week, may have reminded Duffett of the invitation he had received from their mutual friend and banker, David McArthur, to attend the inter-colonial cricket match between Victoria and New South Wales. It was due to start the next day at the Melbourne Cricket Ground. McArthur also happened to be President of the Melbourne Cricket Club and lunch with the President down at the ground was something they had experienced before and enjoyed. It was agreed that they would both go to the match and leave Purves with the run of the library.

The following day was warm and the Melbourne Cricket Ground was bathed in sunshine. The players were resplendent in their creams out on the brilliant green field, surrounded by shady trees which, years before, had been provided by Baron Von Meuller, the creator of Melbourne's beautiful Botanical Gardens. It was a scene more reminiscent of "home" than a Dorothea McKellar one of Australia. A new grandstand had been built two years before. Underneath, it had a dining room, drinks bars, an oyster bar and a fruit stall. It also had the latest in rapid communication, an electric telegraph, which had come to Melbourne early in 1875. Melbournians could now learn about events in Europe and the Americas just 24 hours after their occurrence.

In addition to the new stand there were numerous tents between the trees, all providing a relaxed atmosphere for the large holiday crowd.

However, it was not so relaxing for the Victorian batsmen, who were almost all out before lunch with less than 100 runs. Duffett was pleased with his diversion however, noticing that "Diamond Jim" was soon back to his old-self, moving around with confidence amongst the impressive group gathered for the President's lunch. One of the group, John Cleeland, was well known to Beaney as he was the owner of the very popular Albion Hotel in Bourke Street. Captain Cleeland, an Ulsterman, having been fortunate in the goldfields of California subsequently bought a schooner and traded for some years in the South Pacific before coming to Melbourne and purchasing the hotel. November 1875 saw much celebration at the Albion as his horse, Wollomai, had won the Melbourne Cup. Not all however was smooth sailing in Bourke Street, when some years later Cleeland sued George Watson, the proprietor of a horse and carriage bazaar also in Bourke Street, for publicly calling him a 'dammed scoundrel, a bloody liar and a robber' over a disputed result in a steeplechase. Mr. Aspinall was one of the barristers representing Cleeland, who won the case but was content to have Watson pay just one shilling to the Court. Cleeland would later provide the Cleeland Challenge Cup to the Victorian Cricket Association, to be presented each year to the winner of the interclub competition. It remains with the Melbourne Cricket Club. George Watson, incidentally, was recognised as one of the colony's best horse riders and was a founding member of the Victorian Racing Club and the Melbourne Hunt.

Drinks continued after the lunch even though the players were back on the field. Beaney struck up a conversation with the Hon. John Robertson, the recently re-appointed Premier of New South Wales, who had come down ostensibly on inter-colonial matters, but had found it a convenient opportunity to see some of the traditional match. Robertson was actually elected Premier five times and there is a statue of him in the Sydney Domain. Knowing that New South Wales had the great batsman Bannerman in its side, the Premier wagered loudly that New South Wales would make over 200 runs and as the champagne continued Beaney took up his challenge with a £10 bet, a very large amount for those times.

Victoria was finally dismissed, not long after the luncheon interval, for 136 runs. Bannerman did do well, making 83 for New South Wales. However, at the close of play they were all out for 171, as a young Victorian left arm fast bowler, named Frank Allan, took six wickets for 66 runs. Allan came from Warrnambool and it was said that he developed his strong shoulders throwing boomerangs with the Aborigines in his local district. He, along with Bannerman, would later play for Australia when the 'Test' matches against England began. Winning the bet capped a good day for Beaney.

Meanwhile the assiduous Purves had arrived at Beaney's house early that morning and was pleased to note that Beaney had done his homework. Not only had he left Purves with a very full description of events but also on Beaney's desk were more than a dozen books, each marked in several places by one of Beaney's elaborate appointment cards. Purves noted that in a section of the library there were around twenty books written by Beaney himself. What would have surprised Purves was the subject matter and content of some of these. Whilst *Contributions to the Practice of Conservative Surgery* and *Diseases of the Hip Joint* appeared in keeping with Beaney's position as a prominent surgeon, others such as *Syphilis – its Nature and Diffusion* and *The Generative System* and their content surprised him as some passages, particularly in the latter volume, were little better than pornographic. It is likely that Beaney was encouraged to write this type of literature (in addition to surgical texts), by his publisher, Bailliere, to satisfy and cash in on the public's desire for knowledge about sexually transmitted diseases, which were rife in the gold rush community and in the bustling urban development, then growing with limited control of interpersonal behaviour. These books were all published before 1874 and it was said that they were due to Beaney's immense desire for fame and Balliere's equally immense desire for money.

Purves worked all day on the information Beaney had supplied, sustained only by coffee, and, alternately, water. Although he was not £10 richer when he finished his day, he was confident that he was armed with sufficient information to question the most prominent of medical men on the operation of lithotomy, its variations and its complications. He took a number of the textbooks with him as he left, leaving a note for Dr. Beaney, itemising the ones taken.

It had been the technical aspects of medicine that led Purves to originally enroll in medicine at Trinity College Cambridge in 1861, but he subsequently switched to law, which perhaps offered a greater opportunity for his gifts of expression and persuasion. During the years of his study at Lincolns Inn he successfully supported himself as a literary critic, his writing being well regarded. Besides, the adversarial nature of the court activities suited his personality well.

In the early morning of Tuesday December 28th, a summer storm had hit Melbourne. It was accompanied by thunder and lightening, and it was still raining when Beaney came down for breakfast. There would be no play at the ground that day. If the day was dark, again it was the *Argus* that made it even darker. In it was a letter to the Editor from a George Plant, who ran the Peacock Inn on Rucker's Hill in Northcote. Plant had seen the letters to the paper before Christmas and was writing about the death of his own son, under Beaney, assisted by surgeons Gillbee and Blair (an Alfred Hospital surgeon). He complained that Beaney did not see his child for 48 hours after operating, at which time he had only ordered brandy for the boy, who died about ten hours after the visit. In his letter Plant recounted two other deaths in which he believed Beaney had some involvement. Beaney was affronted by this further exposure but was also concerned that some of the soon to be sworn in jurymen at the inquest might have had their *Argus* delivered that morning. He had met George Plant in the hospital and it was not a pleasant experience. Plant was a solidly built Yorkshire man with a manner he, himself, might regard as blunt and straightforward but to the recipient or observer it was often aggressive. He not only owned the Peacock Inn but also a great deal of land in Northcote, which he rented out to various industries and he had influence also as a local Shire Councillor. Records showed him to be a very outspoken member at meetings, particularly on issues that threatened the maintenance and development of his own interests in that area of Melbourne. He was certainly anti-doctor. In the daily press that year he had objected to paying anything to Dr. McInerny, a local physician, who was appointed early in 1875, at £10 a year, to attend to the district's offensive sights and smells. Both of these insults to the senses abounded in Northcote, as they did in Collingwood, particularly from the slaughterhouses and various establishments, which boiled down pigs and other animals, for the soap and candle industry. Beaney concluded that it would be best under the circumstances not to take part in a war of correspondence with this man, but to let things lie and to concentrate on the case in hand. He spent the rest of that morning checking that he had not overlooked any important elements about stone surgery and its difficulties and dangers, which might justify his actions and assist Purves in his preparations. He found no new information.

By afternoon the storm clouds had cleared and his wife, as a further distraction, persuaded him to accompany her to Emerald Hill (South Melbourne). Whilst she bathed in the shallows inside the new sea baths Beaney took a solitary stroll along the foreshore, possibly rehearsing what he might say if Purves changed his mind and called him to give evidence. For whatever reason Beaney was lost in his thoughts for so long he forgot that his wife would be waiting for him back at the baths. In compensation he accompanied her on an evening shopping venture in the newly gas-lit Clarendon Street, which by then was well known for its fruit and vegetable produce, but even more so for its many skilled dressmakers.

6. The inquest

The inquest commenced on the Wednesday morning at the morgue, then situated near Princes Bridge, on the corner of Swanston and Flinders Streets. The building had been erected in 1871 and served the city until 1888. This prominent location was chosen for a number of reasons, chief among which were that it was close to the Yarra River, from which so many bodies were recovered, and to Swanston Street police station. Before its establishment, bodies used to be stored in hotels, the licensees being paid £1 a body and inquests used to be held at the hotels. Melbourne was ahead of London and New York in establishing its morgue. The only precedent for a purpose-built facility was La Morgue, established in Paris in the 1860s. The fact that Melbourne was ahead of London and New York is probably less indicative of good foresight and planning than it is of a level of need, through lawlessness and a great variance in wealth distribution, in the rapidly growing community.

The Coroner, Dr. Youl, presided at the inquest. Inspector Green, Sub-Inspector Secretan (who three years later would be chasing Ned Kelly) and Detectives Duncan and Gould were present for the Crown. Mr. Purves, being instructed by Mr. Duffett, appeared on behalf of Dr. Beaney.

The men of the jury having been sworn in, the Coroner then addressed them on the background of the case, being an inquiry as to the cause of death of Robert Berth at the Melbourne Hospital on December 5th 1875. He then went on to outline that Berth had a bladder stone for which he underwent an operation on December 2nd. The Coroner stated that following the patient's burial nothing was heard of the matter until roughly ten days later. Then, in connection with another inquest, some disconcerting correspondence appeared in the papers and a particular letter in the *Argus* of December 20th, signed A Practical Surgeon called the attention of the Minister for Justice to the manner of Berth's death. He outlined briefly the police inquiry that then occurred, leading to the exhumation of the body. He was honest enough to indicate that Mr. Barker and Dr. Neild, who together performed the postmortem, had not been his first choices for the task, given the constraints of the holiday period. Nevertheless he believed their qualifications, experience and positions at the University provided reassurance that the autopsy would be appropriately conducted. He would have known, but did not add, that Mr. Beaney had replaced Mr. Barker in election to the Melbourne Hospital earlier in the year.

Whilst Richard Youl prided himself on his honesty and integrity on the bench, others saw him as too rigid. Born in Van Diemans Land, he graduated in medicine in 1842 and obtained an M.D. at St. Andrews

University, in 1844. After studying in Paris and working in Edinburgh and London he had returned to Melbourne in 1850 and started a practice in Flinders Street, later moving to Collins Street. He was appointed Acting Coroner in 1854 and would spend some 30 years presiding over the enormous number of twelve thousand inquests. He is credited with introducing formal medico-legal procedures, including the performance of a post-mortem in every case that came before him. Other achievements concerned the introduction of safety conditions on building sites and sanitary improvements in public institutions. He had a large family of eleven offspring and hated to see children, when sent to prison, having to be housed with adult prisoners. However he also felt that those parents, who could not control their own children, should be punished and that many mothers were not fit for their role. He was in favour of flogging and thought that the death penalty was a kindness. By 1875 he had begun to see a number of cases of death from infection, believed to have been acquired in the hospital and he was building up a feeling of disfavour regarding the Melbourne Hospital. Although he kept this to himself for many years it eventually became public, and Youl was, perhaps unfairly, blamed for the subsequent community reaction against the Melbourne Hospital.

Once, several years on, that community reaction resulted in a riotous mob gathering around a carriage outside the hospital gates, demanding to know why patients were dying in that institution. Inside the carriage, puffing on a cigar was James Beaney. Being hardened against crowd reaction by his previous experiences, Beaney refused to answer them. Instead he is reported to have stubbed out his cigar and exclaimed in a loud voice 'Dreadful lot', dismounted and stepped right through the crowd, into the hospital grounds without being assaulted.

After explaining the circumstances of the postmortem Dr. Youl then invited the jury to view the body, which was lying in an adjoining room at the morgue. Having endured that most unpleasant experience (the body was then about three weeks post-mortem) several members of the jury requested a break and some fresh air. They were granted fifteen minutes outside the building before they were reseated in the hearing room and the examination of witnesses commenced.

The first of the witnesses was Dr. James Edward Neild, a lecturer in forensic medicine at the University Medical School since 1865 and occasional hospital pathologist. He was a red-headed Yorkshire man with a fiery temperament to match. Surprisingly, however, his real interest lay in the theatre. He was a drama critic and his lectures were said to be liberally interspersed with Shakespearian anecdotes, delivered in slow and sonorous speech for dramatic effect. He wrote under several names – 'Christopher Sly', 'Jacques' and 'Tahite', although why he did so is unclear. He helped establish the Victorian branch of the British Medical Association and at one time was editor of the *Australian Medical Journal,* now the *Medical Journal of Australia (MJA).* He claimed in later years that it was he who recognised how good a singer Dame Nellie Melba was and encouraged her to forget her studies and concentrate on a career in opera. Dr. Neild was also known to have publicly stated, concerning some of the questionable books put out by Beaney, that 'It was a class of literature which honourable men shun'.

Dr. Neild read his evidence, which by and large corresponded to the written report of Dr. Fisher, with some small differences. Neild mentioned the presence of some 'dirty reddish-greasy fluid' in the pelvis, a portion of which was removed for later examination. Neild described the surgical incision in the rectum as a tear two inches in length, with black and sloughy edges. He described the left kidney as being of a deep claret colour and the right kidney as being highly congested. The left ureter (tube carrying urine from the kidney to the bladder) he found to be congested at its entrance into the bladder and the right ureter intensely congested along its whole length. The prostate gland (which sits below the bladder in the male) was not visible to him. He stated that the body parts were examined again on the following day by Dr. Barker, Dr Williams, a resident physician, and himself.

He indicated that there was no wound in the abdominal cavity but the peritoneal membrane (smooth layer over the intestines) was exceedingly congested and parts of the neck of the bladder, the prostate and the urethra (voiding tube), were destroyed. Examination of the fluid taken out of the pelvis was found, under the microscope, to contain oil globules, blood corpuscles and pus cells.

Dr. Neild produced two stones, which had been taken from the right kidney at the subsequent examination and some fragments of stone, which had been taken from the bladder. He concluded his written evidence with:

> I believe the cause of death to have been shock from injuries received during an operation, with consequent inflammation of the bladder, ureters and kidneys and peritonitis [inflammation of the abdominal cavity].

Dr. Neild was then questioned by the Coroner about the portion of his statement that indicated that parts of the bladder, part of the urethra and also the prostate gland, were destroyed.

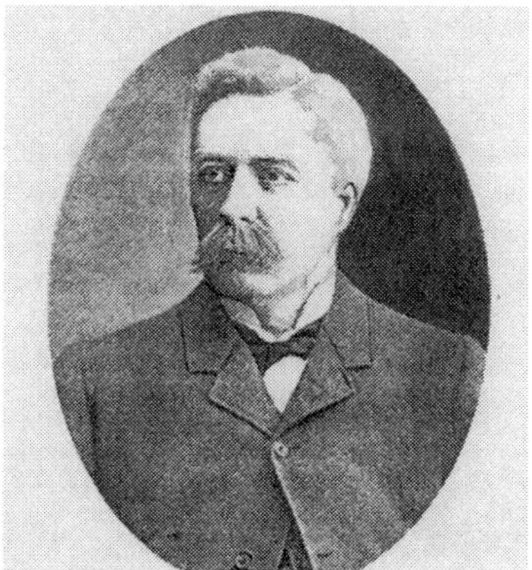

Figure 11: James L. Purves

Dr. Neild replied that they were not present despite a search being made for them. He said from the condition of the parts that remained they appeared to have been removed by violence. At this statement there was a loud call of 'nonsense' from Mr. Beaney. Duffett tugged his arm to caution him, following which Beaney was heard to grumble 'ignorant man'. The coroner cautioned Mr. Beaney against any further such utterances during proceedings.

Dr. Neild was then cross-examined by Mr. Purves, who asked him if he had any practical experience of the operation of lithotomy and of lithotrity

Dr. Neild replied that he had no practical experience of either operation but had seen them performed and understood the former to be cutting a stone out and the latter to refer to crushing a stone.

Dr. Neild was then asked what he considered to be the greatest danger in the operation of cutting for stone and he replied that there were many. Purves sharply requested that he answer the question as to which was the greatest danger and Dr. Neild responded equally sharply that he was not prepared to say what was the greatest but added again that there were many.

Mr. Purves asked if he would call it a grave and serious operation and Dr. Neild responded that there was no question that it was. Purves loudly repeated the witness's last words, 'No question it was grave and serious!'

Q. Is the gravity dependent upon the size of the stone?

A. It is influenced by the size but not altogether dependent.

Q. To a great extent?

A. Yes to a great extent.

Q. It is an operation of grave difficulty?

A. No doubt.

Q. If kidney disease existed at the time of the operation would that increase the danger?

A. Yes! It would be a source of complications.

Mr. Purves asked if Dr. Neild had heard of the disease called surgical kidney and Dr. Neild replied that he had no experience of it but had read of it in text books.

Mr. Purves then asked if the finding of calculi in the right kidney indicated the presence of active disease and Dr. Neild responded that that was not necessarily so.

Q. Are you saying that a healthy kidney may have stones within it?

A. Yes!

Q. Then in your opinion a calculus in a kidney is not a disease at all?

A. I did not say so, the calculus represents a kind of disease itself but the kidney may show no disease.

Mr. Purves then asked if stones could give rise to inflammation, to which Dr. Neild responded that they could give rise to congestion of the kidney.

Q. Would congestion of the kidney be a disease, in your opinion?

A. There are many kinds of disease. I should not call congestion of the kidney an organic disease.

Q. But a congested kidney is not in its natural state?

A. No!

Q. Using the word disease in its broader sense would you say that a highly congested kidney would be a diseased kidney?

A. In its broadest sense, Yes!

The witness by this stage appeared to be having more than a little difficulty in controlling his responses. This was certainly not missed by Purves who turned to the jury and in feigned exasperation proclaimed, 'Well then, we can say that inflammation or congestion of the kidney is a disease'. Before Dr. Neild had a chance to make a further comment Purves turned back to the witness and continued.

Q. In the case of a patient with a diseased kidney would you adopt lithotomy or lithotrity? That is would you cut or crush?

A. Lithotomy is safer.

Purves loudly repeated 'Lithotomy is safer!'

The Coroner intervened and asked if the witness would favour cutting rather than crushing a stone under ordinary circumstance and Dr. Neild replied that if he were the operator, which he did not profess to be, he would prefer to cut rather than to crush a stone. The Coroner then motioned to Purves to continue.

Mr. Purves asked the witness if he knew for how long congestion of the left kidney had been present. Dr. Neild responded that it was probably a matter of several days. Mr. Purves then asked Dr. Neild if he knew that the late Emperor Napoleon III died of "surgical kidney", which is thought to be a flare-up of inflammation in the kidney following surgery or instrumentation of the lower urinary tract.

Dr. Neild again sharply responded that there was a good deal of doubt as to from what Napoleon III had died. Mr. Purves seized on this response and continued questioning:

> Q. Do you admit that there may be a doubt in the minds of the most skilled doctors as to the cause of death following surgery?
>
> A. Yes! Certainly there may.
>
> Q. Even your opinion as to the cause of Robert Berth's death may be fallible?
>
> A. I never saw the deceased during life and therefore I can only give an opinion on the postmortem appearances.
>
> Q. But, given that even the greatest authorities differed on so important a case as that of the late Emperor Napoleon, you will not attempt to say that your opinion is infallible?
>
> A. I would not like to say that anything I stated was infallible, but I have no reason to doubt the correctness of what I have stated in evidence.

> Q. You are satisfied with your own judgement but you will not deny it is fallible?

A. I have taken special pains to satisfy myself on this matter.

Neild's agitation was increasing and Purves, warming to his task, turned to the jury and then back to the witness, picking up a journal as he did so.

Let me quote from a *Lancet* article headed "Surgical Kidney".

It says

> In the report of the post-mortem examination of the body of the Emperor Napoleon III, it is stated that disease of the kidneys existed to a degree which was not suspected, and, if it had been suspected, could not be ascertained.

Commenting upon this in an editorial the *Times* says:

> A man may still, it appears, die under the hands of the finest doctors in the world of a great organic disease, without their knowing anything about it. Unfortunately we have to plead guilty to this charge, but there is much that may be said in mitigation of sentence. The practical surgeon knows only too well.

> Q. Do you now agree that this case, Robert Berth's, is one for a surgeon and not a physician?

A. I am not giving an opinion as a surgeon but one derived from the post-mortem examination. That is my duty. Dr. Barker and others can give evidence as to the surgical part of the case. I only tell you what I saw from the post-mortem.

Q. Do you agree that a certain proportion of operations performed on the urinary organs, even the simplest one of all, such as passing a catheter, may prove fatal from the inflammation of the kidneys?

A. Yes! I have no doubt of that.

Q. Do you agree that you cannot predict with any confidence when such an event may occur?

A. Yes! I agree.

Q. As there were two stones embedded in the right kidney, do you deny that there might have been some inflammation in the kidney?

A. That is possible but you had better state facts instead of surmises.

Q. Are you saying that your opinions are not surmises?

A. I have made no surmises. The post-mortem appearances are facts.

Q. Then the cause of death is not a surmise?

A. It is a logical conclusion from the facts I observed.

Q. This article on surgical kidney states that 'a kidney with chronic irritation requires only a slight additional irritation to rouse it and start changes incompatible with life.' Do you agree with this?

A. Undoubtedly, but this man had wounds in two large organs that were quite sufficient to satisfy my mind that the man may have died from those wounds, apart from anything else.

Q. He "may" have died?

A. Yes!

Purves strode back to his desk to pick up another text repeating the words may have in a loud voice as he did so. He then continued, quoting from a text-

Cooper's *Surgical Dictionary* says:

There is, finally, another cause of death after lithotomy, namely, disease of the kidney and pyelitis; but in most cases it will be found that the operation only hastened death, and has not been its actual cause. However this may be, Mr. Bryant's table shows that pyelitis and inflammation of the kidneys were the cause of death in six out of forty fatal cases. This is a very large proportion, yet not to be wondered at when the condition of many patients labouring under stone is remembered. Bladder calculus seldom exists for any considerable time without producing either disease of the kidneys, or a tendency to disease in these organs, which the slightest exciting cause may light up. Many patients labouring under incipient disease of the kidneys, or with suspicious symptoms are thus operated on and compelled to run a risk which, in the nature of things, it is impossible for them to avoid.

Q. Do you agree with this?

A. Yes! But as a great many people operated upon recover perfectly it is obvious they do not all suffer from fatal disease of the kidney.

Purves asked Dr. Neild if he knew for how many years Berth was suffering from stone disease and Dr. Neild replied that he did not know the patient's history.

Q. Suppose he had been suffering from stone for seven or eight years, and was in and out of hospital because of it, would that in your opinion set up this chronic inflammation of the kidneys you speak about?

A. Knowing that, I am surprised I did not find more disease in the kidneys.

Purves then moved to a more general question and asked whether the body was in a very emaciated state and Dr. Neild replied that the body of the deceased was thin but not emaciated. Purves questioned this response but Dr. Neild held to it.

Q. Would a patient in a weak state having suffered for many years from this disease be at greater risk in an operation of this kind?

A. The longer the man had suffered the more unsuitable he would be for bearing an operation.

Purves paused in his questioning to be sure the jury registered that last response, and then began again.

Q. Now, what operation was it that was performed?

A. I cannot tell you. I was not there.

Q. You pride yourself on your post-mortem experience but assert that you cannot state what the operation was because you did not see it performed?

A. No! Not with the parts all pulled about as they were.

Q. Then you do not know what particular operation was performed in this case?

A. Well, I can only surmise. I should think what is called the median operation, but I examined the body several weeks after burial and the ruin there was, to some of the parts, compels me to speak guardedly on that point.

Q. Was the body in an advanced state of decomposition?

A. Yes! Considerably so, but not so much as to destroy the integrity of those parts that were essential for examination.

Purves asked if Dr. Neild knew for how long the body had been buried and the reply was that he had only just found that it was a period of three weeks.

Purves then asked Dr. Neild how many times he had seen the median operation performed and Dr. Neild's reply was 'possibly four or five times'.

Q. How long is it since the last operation you saw?

A. I suppose about five or six years since.

Becoming extremely agitated Dr. Neild, seeking some support, turned to the Coroner and said 'Sir I believe it is highly irregular to cross-examine me on questions of surgery. Dr. Barker is here for that purpose.'

The Coroner advised Mr. Purves to examine Dr. Neild only on the subject with which he was familiar.

Mr. Purves indignantly retorted 'I submit that my cross-examination is perfectly fair. No man can presume to give evidence as to the real cause of death unless he has fully considered all the surrounding circumstance of the operation itself. Therefore it is important that I test Dr. Neild's knowledge of the actual operation performed.'

Dr. Neild, by now very clearly agitated, loudly protested 'I shall refuse to answer such questions.'

Mr. Purves, extending his arms out with palms up in an exaggerated appearance of bewilderment: 'The gentlemen of the jury are here to determine. the cause of death in this case and you refuse to give evidence, which will assist them to do so?'

Dr. Neild replied 'I refuse to answer any questions which don't relate to the particular duty I was entrusted to perform.'

Mr. Purves, moving close to the witness spoke sharply. 'May I ask who made you a judge of what particular questions you should answer?'

Dr. Neild responded equally sharply. 'I am not a judge, I am a witness and I know what my duties are quite as well as you know yours.'

Mr. Purves said 'Do you know the operation called the median operation?'

Dr. Neild replied 'I shall answer no more questions unless they relate to the post-mortem examination. That is what I was instructed to perform and about which to provide an opinion.'

The Coroner leaned forwards to again intervene. 'I think, Mr. Purves, that you should take the post-mortem appearances from one witness and the surgery from the other. Cross-examine Dr. Neild as far as you choose upon the post-mortem appearances but not upon the surgery. Otherwise you are wasting the time of the jury.'

Mr. Purves, in mock submission, 'I am in your hands, Dr. Youl.'

The Coroner said 'Then we shall proceed so.'

Mr. Purves replied tersely 'Then I shall continue my cross-examination on his own evidence.'

He then asked Dr. Neild about the appearances of the edges of the wound in the perineum. In doing so he held up a coloured plate taken from a textbook of a lithotomy wound. Dr. Neild responded that the wound he noted at the postmortem was much larger and more irregular than the one in the illustration. He agreed with Mr. Purves on further questioning that decomposition of the body would have made a difference to the appearance of the wound, although he insisted that he could tell which tissues were cut and which were torn.

Noting that Dr. Neild had measured the length of the wound at 3 & 7/8 ths inches Mr. Purves asked him what was the length of the wound made in the median operation. Dr. Neild declined to answer, as that was a question on surgery, and not within the scope of his particular function.

Mr. Purves asked him if he had furnished a report to the newspapers about the case including the statement that 'There was a large ragged opening into the bladder nearly 4 inches long and 2 inches wide, which passed down into the rectum and that the prostate gland was found to be torn out to such an extent as to almost escape recognition.'

Dr. Neild refused to respond to any matters except those in his sworn deposition.

Mr. Purves continued questioning on this issue of wound length:

> Q. In that deposition you say 'its length was 3 and 7/8ths inches and its greatest breadth 1 and 3/4 inches?
>
> A. Yes!

Q. Was that the external orifice of the wound?

A. If you read the deposition you will see that I am speaking of the external appearances.

Q. Perhaps you will give me an answer to the question?

A. I will not give you an answer unless you ask me a question that I consider myself bound to reply to. It is no use you bullying me although you may bully other people.

Q. I repeat, was it the external orifice of the wound?

The Coroner intervened indicating that it appeared to be so from the deposition.

Mr. Purves responded that the deposition did not say so and the point he was wishing to make clear to the jury was that if it was the external orifice that Dr. Neild was referring to then it would have been distorted and swollen by decomposition. Turning back to the witness Purves asked him if there was any peritonitis to which the answer was yes.

Purves continued:

Q. Can you explain to the jury what peritonitis is?

A. Peritonitis is inflammation of a membrane that surrounds the bowels and lines the walls of the belly.

Q. Would inflammation of the peritoneum tend to deposit a fluid?

A. Yes! In peritonitis if it is at all advanced, there would be an effusion into the cavity of the belly.

Q. There was no effusion here.

A. I shall need to consult my notes. I do not think it is safe to charge my memory with particulars of this kind.

After a pause to look at his deposition and holding it in trembling hands he responded quietly, 'None whatever!'

One of the jurors, a Mr. Statham, a teacher who had been listening intently, interrupted at this point and asked the Coroner about the "dirty reddish fluid" that had been mentioned earlier and separately examined. Dr. Youl explained to the jury that that small amount of fluid had accumulated during the post-mortem as the organs were being dissected out of the body and had not been there "ab initio".

Purves turned to the jury and forcefully said 'So much for the peritonitis.' Giving the witness no chance to make further comment, he quickly continued his questioning.

> Q. You say the rectum was found to contain hard stools. Before the operation of lithotomy is it proper to clean out the bowels and the rectum?
>
> A. I shall not answer the question. It refers to a matter that is part of the operation and I had nothing to do with the operation.

Purves turned to the Coroner. 'Sir, I ask if a witness is to be allowed to direct the method of his cross-examination?'

The Coroner replied 'I have already advised you, Mr. Purves, that Dr. Neild is called to give evidence as to the post-mortem appearances only and you are examining him as to something else.'

Purves in an exasperated tone asked 'Am I not allowed to cross-examine him on his own evidence? Well then, I am tongue-tied. However, I shall continue.'

> Q. Was there a cut in the rectum?'
>
> A. No! None that I discovered.
>
> Q. There was no cut in the rectum?
>
> A. None that I observed.

Q. In the median operation is there not always a cut into the rectum?

A. I refuse to answer the question. You are wasting your own time, the time of the jury and my time too.

Q. Are you acquainted with the operation known as Lloyd's operation for stone?

The Coroner again intervened 'That is a question of surgery.'

Purves said 'I respectfully beg to differ as it is not a technical question of surgery, but of knowledge only. I asked Dr. Neild if he knows of the existence of a particular operation.'

Exasperated, Dr. Neild answered 'I know a great many things but I am not going to state them here!'

Mr. Purves then picked up yet another textbook, this one by a Dr. Erichsen and read from it to Dr. Neild. The passage he read was a very long one but it essentially stated that in the median operation the prostate is almost always torn, but the tearing is not dangerous unless the capsule of prostate is ruptured as well, for then the urine, which flows through the prostate gland during micturition, can escape into body tissues.

At the end of this reading the Coroner intervened again, with some impatience, 'You can make a speech to the jury Mr. Purves after the evidence is closed and you may then quote from any authority you like. I have given you considerable latitude but it is of no use to ask the witness questions upon a matter which he knows nothing about.'

Purves replied, 'If Dr. Neild says he knows nothing about it I will be satisfied.'

The Coroner said, 'That is what he has said.'

'I beg your pardon!' the witness interjected hotly.

'Then you do know but you refuse to give me the information I seek?' said Purves.

'Yes, I do!' replied Neild, almost shouting.

'Do you consider it comes within the scope of your function to give an opinion as to the cause of death?' said Purves.

A. That is what I am asked to do.

Q. Then that is in within you functions?

A. Always!

Q. Can you state how many immediate causes of death there are following the operation of lithotomy and what they are?

A. I am not going to do that. You are again referring to an operation which I did not see and had nothing to do with. There are a number of gentlemen here who were present at the operation and they will give you every piece of information you can possibly require.

Q. How do you know that?

A. Because I have communicated with them.

Q. Have you communicated with Dr. Barker?

A. He was with me when I made the post-mortem examination.

Q. Have you communicated with him since?

A. Certainly.

Q. And have you seen all of the gentlemen who are going to be witnesses?

A. Some of them.

Q. Have you given them as much information as you have given the jury?

A. I have given them all the information I could.

Mr. Purves then asked Dr. Neild if he had seen the stone which was removed and whether or not it was a large or a small one, and got the reply that he had not seen it and knew nothing of its size.

> Q. Do you say there was any wound in the peritoneum?
>
> A. I think you have asked me that three times. I have stated there was no wound in the peritoneum. It will be next week before the inquest is over if you go on at this rate.

Not wishing to test the patience of the coroner any further Purves indicated that he had no further questions to put to Dr. Neild. The witness, with an obvious feeling of considerable relief, then stood down.

The next witness was Mr. Edward Barker, FRCS, who was lecturer in surgery at Melbourne University and as mentioned before had been replaced by Beaney on the honorary surgical staff at the recent hospital elections. He prided himself on his surgical skills, which had been acknowledged by respected colleagues such as Thomas Fitzgerald, and he deeply felt the injustice of his failure to gain the reappointment. He had come out to Melbourne in the 1840s and although he had a surgical diploma from London he and his brother initially purchased and worked some land in the Westernport region of Victoria. In 1844 his short temper had led him to fight a duel with his neighbour Maurice Meyrick, over an issue about stripping trees. He, in a humane gesture, fired in the air but Meyrick aimed at him, the ball luckily whistling past his ear.

Barker also ventured into gold mining in the Mount Alexander fields when the rush began but he didn't last long in that pursuit, and returned to Melbourne and the Melbourne Hospital in 1862.

The Coroner asked if Mr. Barker had been present at the operation performed on Robert Berth, and the witness advised that he was not there, but that he was present at the post-mortem examination of the body and that he did the "cutting part". The Coroner asked if the witness agreed with Dr. Neild's evidence, including the measurements of the wounds described. He did. The Coroner then requested the witness to advise the jury on the different types of cutting operations that there were for stone. Barker described the lateral operation as the commonest and that there were three versions of it, as there were for the median operation, the one known as Lloyd's involving an extension of the incision into the rectum. He also advised that there was an operation done for large stones by which the bladder is opened from in front, above the pubis (the midline bony prominence at the lower end of the abdomen), called the suprapubic operation. Barker stated that he was the first in the colony to use Lloyd's method. He stated that the object of the median operation was to avoid cutting or tearing through the prostate gland.

All of this evidence, as Purves noted, was given with a great air of self-assurance. The Coroner then produced the stone, which had been in Berth's bladder and asked if it was possible to extract that stone without considerable injury to the soft parts, by any of the operations from below. Barker responded that it would be utterly impossible but that it could be done by the suprapubic operation or might be done from below by crushing the stone. With these responses the Coroner's interest appeared to quicken and he followed up more directly.

Q. Is that the usual practice?

A. It is the usual practice and has been adopted numerous times.

Q. It is possible to ascertain the size of a stone before you proceed to operate?

A. It is easy. It should be done always.

At this response Mr. Beaney rose to intervene, but receiving a "look" and a shake of the head from Purves he sat down without speaking.

The Coroner continued,

Q. It is easy to ascertain the size of a stone in the bladder?

A. Yes! Before either cutting or otherwise.

Q. And it should be done before an operation is commenced?

A. Yes!

Q. Is it more dangerous to tear the soft parts, than to cut them?

A. A great deal more.

One of the jurymen, a tradesman called McDonald interrupted at that stage. 'Do we understand the witness to say that the stone produced here could have been crushed?'

The Coroner replied, 'I did not ask him specifically as to this stone but I shall do so.'

Barker responded before the question was put. 'I should certainly think there would be no difficulty in breaking this stone up.'

Mr. Beaney could be heard to whisper in a not too quiet voice to Duffett, 'I tried and it could not be done.'

The Coroner continued.

Q. It could be easily crushed?

A. I believe so.

The Coroner then invited Mr. Purves to cross-examine.

Q. I suppose you have had a large experience as a surgeon.

A. I was eight years in a hospital at home before I came here and have been twenty-five years a surgeon to the Melbourne Hospital.

Beaney could again be heard whispering to Duffett-, 'He is not there now!'

Purves continued.

Q. How many times have you performed the operation of lithotomy with the median operation?

A. I suppose I have performed it forty times at least.

Q. How many times have you performed the particular operation known as Lloyd's?

A. I dare say I have performed Lloyd's operation five and twenty times. As I said I was the first to do it in the colony.

Q. Have you ever had the misfortune to lose a patient?

A. Yes!

Q. How many patients have you lost?

The witness shifted a little uncomfortably.

A. I think my average is about one in six. That is a very fair average.

Q. What has been the most frequent cause of death in your cases?

A. I think I may say that in all it has been peritonitis.

Q. Do you recognise lithotomy as one of the most dangerous operations known to surgery?

A. I do not.

Q. Then you consider that one death in six is not a higher average than in the usual run of operations?

A. In amputation through the thigh the average is about one in three and a half.

Q. Is there any other operation from which there is a higher average of deaths than there is from lithotomy?

A. Plenty.

Q. What others?

A. There is tracheotomy, the surgical opening of the main windpipe.

Q. I suppose that the patient in that case is always on the verge of death. Is not one death in five or six a high average in the ordinary range of surgical operations?

A. No! It is in certain operations.

Q. In your opinion is the presence of a calculus or calculi in the kidney a disease of the kidneys?

A. No! I don't call it a disease of the kidney. There are plenty of people who have passed calculi and enjoyed good health afterwards.

Q. Then a kidney may have a stone in it and yet be healthy?

A. There may be a little irritation but it does not follow that there is disease of the kidney.

Q. Have you ever known calculi in the kidney to cause death?

A. I have, but there must be other disease with it.

Q. Would a kidney having calculi in it, like those produced in this case, be prone to inflammation like a smouldering fire that might be lit up in a moment?

A. No! I don't think so.

Q. Is pyelitis or inflammation of the kidney a disease likely to assume serious proportions after the operation of lithotomy?

A. I have yet to know what the symptoms were that this man suffered from after the operation before I can answer that question.

Purves looked at the jury and then back at the witness and asked with feigned surprise.

Q. You know nothing about it?

A. No!

Q. Will you describe what appearances the left kidney presented?

A. It was a crimson colour, the vessels were all injected with blood and as far as I could see it was in an active state of inflammation.

Purves, pausing then to let the witness's last comment admitting the presence of active inflammation in the left kidney sink in, chose another medical textbook from the collection and showed it to the witness. It was by a Dr. William Caulson and the witness agreed that he was an authority.

Mr. Purves then read out a long list of the causes of death after lithotomy, the commonest causes being shock and disease of the kidneys, although the list also included peritonitis.

Purves asked if Mr. Barker recognised these as causes, which must of necessity be met within a surgeon's practice. Barker accepted that it was so but went on to state that that particular edition of the book was out of date and that in a later edition Caulson wrote of the use of a lithotrite, being introduced through an incision in the perineum, to break up stones

Purves asked:

> Q. Where are those cases to be found?
>
> A. I cannot say where, but I know they are to be found.
>
> Q. Have you seen any done?
>
> A. No! I have not.

Purves turned to the jury and shrugged his shoulders in a gesture suggesting doubt as to the veracity of

Barker's statement about such a procedure. He went on:

> Q. Can you say how long Berth had the disease of the kidney before he died?
>
> A. I should say the disease of the left kidney was quite recent.
>
> Q. Supposing chronic inflammation of the kidneys existed, would an operation necessarily tend to increase that inflammation and augment that disease?
>
> A. Decidedly, but in that case there should be no operation.

The Coroner intervened again with a question.

> Q. If chronic inflammation of the kidney existed at the time of the operation it would be liable to become acute?
>
> A. Yes, it would be liable to become acute!

Mr. Purves again allowed time for that response to be received by the jury, then picking up yet another textbook addressed the witness again.

> Q. Dr. Humphrey, the celebrated Cambridge surgeon, records a case of great interest in which although little force was used the bladder was

ruptured by the forceps and the stone escaped through the laceration into the peritoneal cavity. Suppose chronic inflammation of the kidneys was present, would such an accident as the one I described augment it?

A. Certainly it would.

Q. Is it possible that such an accident as that could have happened with you operating?

A. Yes, if the bladder was in a diseased state, but not if it wasn't.

Q. Do you consider yourself a more able surgeon than Dr. Humphrey?

A. I don't know, I have had a pretty good experience.

Q. Are you saying that it could not happen to you, that you might accidentally rupture the bladder in extracting a stone?

A. It would not.

Purves raised his eyebrows and again turned to the jury to indicate his surprise at this surgeon's self-confidence then continued.

Q. Returning to the median operation, after you have made the incision what have you to do next?

A. You must dilate.

Q. Does dilatation, in ordinary language, mean stretching?

A. Certainly it does, but not tearing.

Q. Do you regard Erichsen as an authority and do you use his writing in your University lecturing?

A. I do.

Mr. Purves picked up a textbook from which he had previously read and returned with it to the witness, to confirm its authorship.

Q. Now listen to what Erichsen says as to dilatation: "So, in the median operation, the prostate may be dilated to a considerable extent without opening into its capsule. I have used the word 'dilate,' but dilatation appears to me to be an erroneous term. I believe that the prostate is not simply dilated, but partially lacerated." You say it is never lacerated?

A. You asked me about the bladder. I never said anything of the kind about the prostate gland. I said I would not do it if I could help it.

Q. Do you agree with this description of dilatation?

A. In any cases where I have had the opportunity of making a post-mortem examination, I have not lacerated the prostate. I mean in cases in which I have operated upon the living subject and the patient has afterwards died.

Mr. Purves murmured audibly, whilst turning the pages of the same text, 'Your patient died afterwards,' and then more loudly

Q. Listen to Erichsen again: "Manipulation of the Forceps and Extraction of the Stone – In the adult, the main difficulty of lithotomy does not lie in entering the bladder, but in the completion of the operation – that for which the operation has been undertaken – the removal of the stone. And the difficulty and danger increase in proportion to the size of the calculus." Do you agree with this?

A. Yes.

Q: Erichsen goes on to say "The tissues between the neck of the bladder and the perineal integuments must either be widely cut or extensively torn and bruised to allow the passage of a large stone." Do you agree with this?

A. Yes but it is not necessarily so, there is, as I stated earlier, another edition of Erichsen's work, which was published last year.

Replacing the textbook Purves moved to pick up the stone, which was now an exhibit, and returned with it to the witness.

Q. Is the calculus that was extracted in this case a large one?

A. It is.

Q. Have you ever seen so large a stone?

A. Yes!

Q. Where?

A. There was a much larger one removed at Geelong.

Q. Was that not after death?

A. There was one removed after death but there was a much larger one, than the one in this case, removed whilst the patient was living.

Purves put down the stone and returned to the Erichsen text from which he had been quoting. He read a long passage about the difficulties encountered in the median operation, particularly at the neck of the bladder. The passage ended with a caution about the danger of an accidental rupture of the bladder.

Q. Do you admit there may be dangerous and fatal accidents?

A. I certainly do.

Q. Do you agree with this further statement from Erichsen that in the median operation, with a large stone the bladder may be injured?

A. I disagree with Mr. Erichsen because I believe you can take out a larger stone by the median operation – by Lloyd's operation – than you can by the lateral.

The Coroner intervened, 'That is only your opinion?'

A. That is my opinion.

Mr. Purves went on.

Q. How can you determine the size of a stone in the bladder?

A. In the first place you can tell it pretty well by using a sound, but if you cannot determine it that way you can always introduce an instrument by which you can measure it.

The Coroner intervened again. 'There is an instrument by which you can measure a stone in the bladder?'

A. Yes!

Mr. Purves continued,

Q. Do you mean to say that is infallible?

A. Yes.

Q. Absolutely?

A. Absolutely infallible.

Q. If the text writers say that the difficulty of lithotomy is intensified where the stone is of unusual size, what do you say to that?

A. I say you should break the stone.

Q. Have you ever made a mistake in judging the size of a stone?

A. I don't know that I have.

Q. Have you?

A. I say that I don't know that I have, at least not where I have measured it.

Q. Have you performed operations without measuring?

A. Certainly I have.

Q. Then you have operated for stone in the bladder without measuring the stone before you operated?

A. Yes but I felt convinced they were small stones. I could tell by the sound as well as possible.

Q. Is it possible for a surgeon to operate for stone and find no stone at all?

A. It has been done.

Q. And by qualified surgeons?

A. Well! I should not call them qualified.

Q. By surgeons?

A. Yes, by surgeons.

Purves returned to the subject of stone crushing.

Q. Do you know what lithotrites there are at the Melbourne Hospital?

A. No! I always took my own instruments when I did any operation.

Purves picked up one of the hospital instruments, held it towards the witness and asked him if he had any objection to looking at the hospital's instruments to which Barker replied that he did not.

Q. Is this a lithotrite?

A. Yes it is a French one I believe.

Mr. Purves looked at the jury.

Q. It happens to be one made by Evans and Wormull, the London firm, which has been making instruments for over two hundred years. Is this what you would use to crush the stone?

A. No.

Q. What would you use?

A. I would use a much more powerful instrument.

Q. Where would you get it?

A. There are plenty of lithotrites stronger than that, I think I have got three.

Q. Is there a stronger one in the hospital?

A. I believe so.

Q. Have you seen it?

A. I have seen several in the hospital.

Q. Have you seen any stronger ones than this?

A. Yes I have.

Q. Would this instrument be the sort of one you would take to crush the stone?

A. Certainly not because I should take a stronger instrument.

Q. These instruments are made to scale are they not?

Dr. Barker was by now more than a little irritated as he tersely replied that he knew they were made to scale and that he did not want to look at the instrument.

Q. What is the scale on this instrument if you know all about it?

A. Those are copied from the French and they are made in 10ths.

Q. This happens to be made in 6ths.

A. (changing his mind, takes the instrument and reads from it) Well, it does not signify whether it is in 10ths or in 6ths.

Q. Does the gauge indicate the crushing capacity of the instrument?

A. No, it indicates the size of the stone.

Q. Then as it is gauged up to one inch and a quarter only it would not be applicable for stones of a large size.

A. Yes.

Q. Do you say the stone extracted from the man Berth could be easily crushed?

A. Yes I believe it could be easily.

Q. Would this lithotrite crush the stone?

A. I have already told you it would not but there are others that will.

Q. How long would it take to crush this stone?

A. I could not say. It might take a minute; it might perhaps take two or three minutes.

At this stage the Coroner intervened, 'Do I understand that at all events a few minutes would be sufficient time for crushing this stone?'

> A. A few minutes would be quite sufficient.

A gruff note of dissent could be heard coming from Beaney's direction.

> Q. How many instruments are there in the stock of the Melbourne Hospital that are stronger than this one?

> A. I should say there are three or four at least. I think there are six lithotrites in the hospital.

The Coronor interrupted Purves, 'You had better examine the officer of the hospital, who has charge of the instruments, for information as to the number.'

Purves, nodding, continued,

> Q. Have you got any lithotrites?

> A. Yes.

> Q. Here with you?

> A. No.

> Q. Do you recognise that in surgery you must use your best judgement on any critical juncture?

A. Certainly you must do that. You must act for the best.

Q. You also recognise that in surgical operations exceptional circumstances may occasionally arise, which will force you to act on the spur of the moment.

A. Yes.

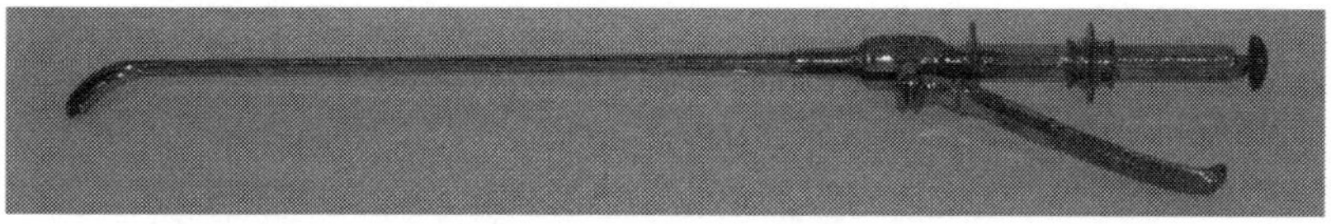

Figure 12: 19th century lithotrite.

Purves let that response linger with the jury and appeared to busy himself with the textbooks, but did not pick one up.

Q. Returning to Lloyd's operation, which cut is made into the rectum?

A. The first incision should go into the rectum.

Q. When the stone is being brought out of the bladder, would the cut in the rectum necessarily be extended if it were a large stone?

A. If it was a large stone it might be extended.

The Coroner intervened, 'The question is whether in the extraction of a large stone the cut in the rectum would be dilated in its passage?'

A. I think it would be by very little.

Q. Surely that is dependent upon the size of the stone?

A. It would depend upon the size of the stone.

Q. In the extraction of a large stone is it not necessary to use great force?

A. No, it is not necessary to use great force, in fact one is always cautioned against it.

The Coroner asked: 'It is not necessary to use great force in extracting a large stone – it should not be done?'

A. It should not be done!

Purves continued:

Q. Will you deny that some amount of traction must be used in extracting a stone from the bladder?'

A. I do not believe in that at all.

Mr. Purves again moved to pick up another textbook *A System of Surgery,* edited by Timothy Holmes and read a long passage from it about the difficulty of extracting a stone and the injuries that may result to both the prostate gland and the bladder when a forceps is used, as the forceps may also enclose a section of either the bladder or the prostate, and, if the operator is unaware of this, a subsequent laceration of either organ may result in extravasation of urine into the body tissues.

Mr. Purves then looked at the witness for a comment.

A. That could happen, but it is avoidable.

Q. Every surgeon has not the calmness and the firm hand of yourself, I suppose?

A. I do not know.

Q. Is it possible for a surgeon to do this damage?

A. It is not generally. I should say no person who would do it is a surgeon.

Q. But this authority calls himself so!

A. I don't care about that.

Before putting the text down Purves showed its front cover with the author's name to the jury as he passed close to them, and said 'Hunterian Professor of Surgery and Pathology at the Royal College of Surgeons, London.' He then turned back to the witness.

> Q. Well, having made the incision and having dilated all the parts and seized the stone, would you then, if you found the stone too large, adopt the suprapubic operation?
>
> A. No, but I should break up the stone, and that is what aught to have been done.

Dr. Beaney had been sitting quietly, for the most part, during this time (remarkably so Duffett may have thought) and was making occasional notes. However at this last statement by Barker he rose to interject again to say that he had tried, but was tugged down by his solicitor, as Purves continued.

> Q. You say it is the easiest thing possible to put in an instrument and crush the stone?
>
> A. It would be if you had the right instrument.
>
> Q. How long would you wait for such an instrument in such an operation?
>
> A. I would expect to have the instruments in the room at the time.

Q. Would you expect them to be in the hospital stock?

A. I should expect them to be in the operating room at the time.

Q. Would you expect them to be in the hospital stock?

A. Certainly I would.

Q. And suppose you were conducting an operation and you asked for this particular stone crusher and it was not there, what would you do?

A. Send for it.

Q. How long would you wait with the patient under chloroform?

A. If he waited half an hour it would be nothing.

Q. Would an hour be anything?

A. I do not know that an hour would signify any danger.

Q. Then the length of time that an operation takes has no bad effect upon the patient?

A. I say keeping the man under chloroform; I don't say the operation.

Q. Keeping the patient under chloroform would have no ill effect upon him?

A. No.

Q. Could you keep a patient an indefinite time under chloroform?

A. You could keep the patient a couple of hours under it without him being injured by the chloroform.

Q. If he was a weak, spare man?

A. Yes that would not make much difference.

Purves again clearly displayed disbelief to the jury at this response, and several heads in the jury nodded also in disbelief, knowing there had been three deaths from chloroform reported in the press in that year. (Incidentally chloroform was produced in John Hood's pharmacy, where Beaney had assisted as a young man). After a pause Purves then continued.

Q. How long does it take you as an experienced surgeon to conduct the median operation from beginning to end?

A. I think it very long if I am three minutes.

Q. What?

A red-faced Mr. Beaney again rose to indicate his disbelief, and this time Duckett had to use both arms to draw him back down to his seat. The latter recognised that a slanging match between the witness and the accused would not please the Coroner and might put the jury offside. Duckett was confident Purves would handle the witness and whispered that message to Beaney.

A. You may look surprised. I consider it very long if I am three minutes.

Q. Over the whole operation?

A. Over the whole operation.

Q. I thought you would take three minutes merely to crush the stone?

A. Three minutes is a long time for the whole operation.

Mr. Beaney could not contain himself and shouted 'It could not be done!'

The Coroner advised Beaney to refrain from further interjecting, warning him that he risked removal from the proceedings. Purves continued.

Q. How long do you take to dilate the parts?

A. I do not take many seconds to dilate the parts.

Q. Then you would tear them roughly asunder?

A. I would not. I do not tear them at all.

Q. Do you think it is an advantage to be only three minutes?

A. I do.

Q. A great advantage?

A. The sooner you get an operation over the better.

Q. How do you reconcile that with the statement that you would think nothing of keeping a patient half an hour after chloroform?

A. I would do so if the circumstance required it.

Purves, shaking his head, moved back to his desk and deliberately and loudly closed the last textbook, from which he had been quoting. The jury might have heard him say sarcastically in a low voice 'No need for world experts when we have our Mr. Barker.'

He returned to the witness.

Q. Have you had a consultation on this matter at your house?

A. No. We had a meeting not a consultation.

Q. Who was present?

A. Dr Williams, Dr. Neild and myself.

Q. Did you advise Dr. Beaney that you were having this private conference at your house?

A. No

Q. He did not know you were going to have this secret conference?

A. It was not a secret conference.

Q. Have you seen any other persons who are to be witnesses in this case?

A. This meeting took place last evening. Dr. Annand was by, but that was all. We were only drawing up the post-mortem appearance and nothing else.

Q. How long did this affair occupy?

A. It may have taken from half an hour to three quarters of an hour.

Q. Did you talk over what you were going to say?

A. No we only talked over the post-mortem appearances.

Purves moved up very close to the witness and asked,

Q. Dr. Barker, have you ever given any instruction, either by yourself or in company with another directly or indirectly, to take legal proceedings against Dr. Beaney?

A. I have not.

Q. With reference to the election of honorary surgeons in the hospital?

The witness reddened. Loudly and angrily he replied 'That has nothing to do with this case.'

Q. I ask you for the facts?

A. I shall not answer you.

Q. That has nothing to do with the case?

A. You have got your answer.

Purves moved back to the exhibit table, picked up the large stone and holding it towards Mr. Barker asked him what sort of stone it was. Barker replied that it was probably a phosphate stone, which is a hard stone, but not as hard as a mulberry one, which is composed of uric acid. On questioning he agreed that some stones are mixed in content and can be harder on the inside than the outside. The questions continued,

Q. Can you say how many years this calculus has been in formation?

A. It might have been very rapidly formed or it might have been formed over a long time.

Q. Might it have been ten years?

A. It might have been.

Q. Suppose it was built up over ten years, would not the interior be materially firmer and harder than any of the exterior portion?

A. Yes, but that would not prevent it being broken up.

Q. Would it increase the difficulty and danger of breaking it?

A. No, it would not.

Q. Not the fact of the centre bit being very hard?

A. Parts of it would be soft but you could easily break it down and so diminish the size of it?

Q. What is the largest stone that you have removed?

A. I cannot say.

Q. Have you seen any surgeon remove a stone of more than two inches in diameter?

A. I cannot say I have.

Purves, picking up another textbook read the following, 'Stone in the kidney or bladder is a not uncommon affection. It is generally a painful one and is often fatal.' He looked at Barker for a response.

'I don't know that it is often fatal,' said Barker. 'It is a painful affection.'

Purves recognised that he wasn't going to gain much ground from pursuing the witness further and indicated to the Coroner that he had exhausted his questioning.

The Coroner advised Mr. Barker that he could stand down and then addressed the court, 'That will conclude the proceedings for today. Tomorrow resident members of the hospital staff will be interviewed, together with others who attended the operation on Robert Berth.' He advised the jurymen that they were to speak to no one about the case in the intervening period.

That evening passers-by in Collins Street might have noticed that the odd stone-shaped artefacts were no longer present in the window of the bookshop at 140 Collins Street. Perhaps they would also have noticed, through the fading evening light, a rather forlorn figure sitting on the upper steps of the Scots church, until beckoned by an anxious woman on the footpath. Beaney was not a regular churchgoer but had struck up a friendship with the Reverend Charles Strong, the Minister of Scots Church, and had gone over to divert his mind from the inquest through dialogue with the minister. Like Beaney he too was a controversial and headstrong character. He recognised the changes taking place in society and in theological argument. He did his best to bring his congregation along with him but his "modern scientific notions" were not well received and they led to his eventual dismissal from the church in 1883.

Strong would have been welcomed however by the young New South Wales group of Presbyterian ministers, who met regularly in that state to discuss experimental theology. They called themselves 'The Heretics'. His views would also have been better tolerated by the members of the Melbourne Unitarian Church, which in 1873 had appointed its first female minister, the Reverend Martha Turner. Both the

Unitarian Church and she were regarded as progressive thinkers and were supportive of opening galleries, libraries and museums on Sundays. The Rev. Strong subsequently established his own church, firstly in Flinders Street and then in Russell Street as his supporters decreased in number. He differed from Beaney in having a deep social conscience however and ministered to the poor in the surrounding suburbs. He established the first crèche in Australia to assist the working mothers of Collingwood. With his wife, who was a nurse, he also organised the first meeting to introduce District Nursing into the colony.

Unfortunately on this particular night that Beaney had sought his companionship, the Rev. Strong was elsewhere lecturing. Beaney's mood, however, may have been soothed by the voices of the Presbyterian Ladies College choir, one of them belonging to Helen (Nellie) Mitchell, as they rehearsed for the coming New Year's Day ceremony.

7. The inquest continues

Melbourne's reputation for changeable weather was true to form and the following day was actually hot and sunny. There were only a few light cirrus clouds, high in the sky. Beaney's mood had improved also with further contemplation of the first day's proceedings. He felt that Purves had done very well with the would-be executioners and was likely to do even better with the junior doctors who were to give evidence on this day. He was also amazed at Purves for his quick grasp of the intricacies of the operation. Furthermore he could not recall marking some of the passages from which Purves had quoted.

The first witness questioned on the second morning was Dr. George Annand, a resident surgeon at the Melbourne Hospital. The name Annand was certainly well known to the hospital as his father, a successful businessman and part owner of the city's first foundry, had been on the Committee of Management for a great many years. This association gave George junior a little more confidence than his knowledge, ability and experience should have allowed.

Dr. Annand was questioned by the Coroner on the identification and age of the deceased and had it confirmed that Mr. Berth was a patient in the Melbourne Hospital, admitted under Mr. Beaney, and had been suffering from a stone in the bladder.

[Surgeons could be referred to as Mr., and the junior staff were always careful to use this term, which was a leftover from the time when barbers did the blood-letting. The Barber Surgeons Guild still exists in the UK to this day, the Company of Barber Surgeons having been founded over 500 years ago.]

Annand indicated that the patient had been in tolerable health, but was suffering from pain with the stone, especially on walking. He indicated that Mr. Beaney saw the patient on November 30th and surgery was arranged for December 2nd. The Coroner then asked

> Q: Did Mr. Beaney examine him when he saw him on the Tuesday November 30th?
>
> A. Yes, he passed a sound into the bladder.
>
> Q. Did he say anything about the stone?
>
> A. No, he simply said he would operate on Thursday, the next operating day.
>
> Q. Was there no consultation?
>
> A. No.
>
> Q. Was there none called?
>
> A. No.

Q. Whose duty is it to call one?

A. It is the honorary surgeon's duty to give directions for the calling of a consultation if he wishes for one.

Q. Is it not imperative, according to the rules of the hospital, that there shall be a consultation before operation?

A. It is.

Q. Do not the rules direct who should call the consultation?

Mr. Purves interrupted, 'You had better have the rules produced if you want to use them.'

'Very well,' the Coroner tersely responded, 'we shall get the rules, which will speak for themselves.'

The Coroner then continued with his questions.

Q. Was the operation done on the day appointed?

A. Yes.

Q. Who was present?

A. Being engaged in assisting I did not notice all who were present. I know the names of some but there were a great many persons there whom I cannot remember.

Q. The operation took place in the presence of a number of persons?

A. Yes.

Q. Who assisted at operation?

A. Mr. Webb, who was one of the assistant honorary surgeons in the hospital.

Q. Were any of the honorary surgeons there beside Mr. Beaney?

A. No.

Q. Chloroform was given to the patient I suppose?

A. Chloroform was administered by the resident physician, Dr. Lewellin.

Q. How long did the operation take?

A. About an hour and a half.

Q. Was much force used in extracting the stone?

A. Yes, a very considerable force.

Duffett quickly cautioned Beaney before he could respond to this.

Q. Was it used by Mr. Beaney exclusively?

A. No, Mr. Beaney and Mr. Webb together levered the stone out.

Q. How do you mean levered it out?

A. One had a lever above the stone and one had a lever below it and they levered it out.

The Coroner motioned the court clerk to hold up some instruments and asked

Q. Are these the instruments?

A. Yes, one is an ordinary scoop and the other a spring scoop.

Q. What length of time did the extraction of the stone occupy?

A. Over an hour.

Q. When difficulties arose as to the size of the stone was there any consultation held as to what should be done?

A. No, suggestions were made, but Mr. Beaney did not consult with anyone.

Q. What suggestion was made?

A. A suggestion was made that the stone should be crushed and extracted piecemeal.

Q. By whom was that suggestion made?

A. By Dr. Moloney and also by Mr. Webb.

Q. Mr. Beaney refused to crush the stone?

A. Yes.

Q. Did he say he would not do it?

A. He said he would like to get it out whole.

Q. You had charge of the patient after the operation?

A. Yes.

Q. What happened to him? Did he recover from the shock?

Dr. Annand stated that for the first 36 hours Mr. Berth seemed to be doing well, was conversing clearly, with no evidence of shock and was not in a great degree of pain. However after that period his condition deteriorated and on the night of December 4th it appeared that peritonitis was setting in. He did not rally from that period and died on December 5th.

The Coroner then motioned to Mr. Purves to cross-examine and Mr. Purves asked Dr. Annand if he knew where the patient had come from. Dr. Annand responded that he knew that Mr. Berth had come from the Amherst Hospital, where he had been for around 18 months, suffering from a stone in the bladder, the stone having been present for three or more years.

Mr. Purves questioned:

> Q. When he was admitted into the Melbourne Hospital what condition was he in?
>
> A. He was not a stout man, but he was in tolerable condition.
>
> Q. Was he not reduced?
>
> A. He was a thin man but he was not what you would call emaciated.
>
> Q. He said he suffered great pain?
>
> A. Yes, on walking.

Q. When Dr. Beaney said he would operate on him did he direct you to do anything?

A. No he gave no directions.

Q. Is it not your business to prepare patients for an operation?

A. Yes it is also the business of the honorary surgeon to give any directions as to what he wishes to be done to the patients before operating.

Q. Is it proper before the operation of lithotomy to clear out the rectum?

A. Yes it is.

Q. Was it done at this stage?

A. I ordered that the patient should have an enema.

Q. Whom did you order?

A. The wards man.

Q. Did you take any steps to see that your order was carried out?

A. (somewhat dismissively) It is not necessary in the Melbourne Hospital.

Q. Have you heard that the enema was not given?

A. I have heard since that it was not. The wards man told me that the reason he did not do it was because the man's bowel had operated freely that day without using an enema.

Q. Did you inform Mr. Beaney that the patient's bowels had operated naturally and that no enema had been given?

A. (less smugly) I did not know it at the time.

Q. Very well, let us move on – Now you say there was no consultation?

A. No.

Q. Do you know whether Mr. Beaney sent notices to the other honorary surgeons that he was about to perform the operation?

A. He directed me to send out notices of the operation but he said nothing about a consultation.

Q. Did you send out the notices?

A. Yes I sent notices to the four honorary surgeons: Mr. James, Mr. Fitzgerald, Mr. Howett and Mr. Beaney himself.

Q. Did any of the other three attend?

A. No, I have stated so already.

Q. Then with whom was Mr. Beaney to consult?

A. Notices of consultations are altogether distinct from notices of operations. They are printed on different cards.

The foreman of the Jury, a Mr. Burton, who was a teacher, interrupted-Is it usual to have consultations?

The Coroner replied, 'The rule of the hospital is distinct upon the subject; it says that no important operation shall be performed, except in an emergency, without a consultation.'

Purves then continued the cross-examination:

Q. How long have you been at the Melbourne Hospital?

A. Nearly three years.

Q. Do you mean to tell the Jury that the rules of the hospital are never broken in any case?

A. I do not suppose that there are any rules that are not broken, neither there or anywhere else.

Q. Are consultations for simple operations necessary?

A. What do you mean by a simple operation?

Q. Cutting a man's leg off for instance?

A. Absolutely necessary.

Q. There are always consultations?

A. As far as I know there are.

Q. In every case?

A. Except in cases of emergency, which did not allow time for consultation.

Q. Why did you not call a consultation in this case?

A. Because I did not receive any directions from the honorary surgeon.

Q. (walking up close to the witness, leaning towards him, and asking quietly) May I ask, do you dislike Dr. Beaney?

A. No.

Q. Dr. Beaney has not been long at the hospital?

A. He has been there three or four months.

Q. Did you tell Dr. Beaney about this inflexible rule?

A. He knows the rules very well.

Q. Did you call attention to it when he told you to send out the notices of operation?

A. It was not my duty.

Q. Then you only do you duty?

A. That is all.

Q. Have you known notices sent out and no attention being paid to them by the honorary surgeons?

A. Do you mean by all of the honorary surgeons or by some of them?

Q. By some.

A. Yes.

Q. Is it not a fact that this patient was sent down specifically from Amherst Hospital to be operated upon for stone?

A. Mr Webb sent him into the Melbourne Hospital for an operation.

Q. Specifically for an operation for stone?

A. Yes.

Q. Well then why should there be a consultation if he was sent into the hospital to be operated upon for stone, if the operation had been determined upon before he came there?

A. He was sent in by Mr. Webb to be cut for stone. That is all I can say.

Q. (loudly) Very well, it is clear that he was sent to the Melbourne Hospital to have an operation for stone. Now let us move to after the operation. You say the patient improved after the operation?

A. I say he went on well.

Q. When symptoms of peritonitis showed themselves, was it your business to treat them?

A. Yes I am in charge in the absence of Mr. Beaney.

Q. Did you take steps to treat the peritonitis?

A. I did.

Q. Did Mr. Beaney see the patient?

A. He saw him in the morning after the operation at which time the patient had no symptoms of peritonitis. Mr. Beaney saw him again on the afternoon of December 5th and by then the peritonitis was well marked.

Q. What did the patient die from?

A. The symptoms he had were—

Q. (interjecting) Tell me what he died from first and then describe the. symptoms afterwards.

A. I can only give my opinion from the symptoms.

Q. Tell me your opinion first and provide the symptoms afterwards. What did the man die from?

A. Peritonitis.

Q. (seizing on it, turning to the jury) But from the post-mortem we have no evidence of peritonitis. (turning back to a rather nervous Dr. Annand) Dr. Annand, with your experience, can you detect the disease called "surgical kidney" by any symptoms?

A. I don't know that I could unless the symptoms were very well marked.

Q. If this man had diseased kidneys could you detect it?

A. Do you mean surgical disease?

Q. Surgical disease of the kidney.

A. No, I could not.

Q. (pausing) You arrived at your verdict of peritonitis from external symptoms?

A. From symptoms during life and immediately preceding death.

Q. If you were told that one kidney was in a violent state of inflammation, congested throughout all its tissues, would that affect your verdict in any way?

A. (hesitantly) I should then say that he died of peritonitis and inflammation of the kidneys.

Q. Now Dr. Annand, we have already been shown that at postmortem there was no evidence of peritonitis, so let us concentrate on the kidneys. Is not an operation on a patient who has a diseased kidney, or a tendency to diseased kidney, almost equivalent to "stirring the fire?"

A. Yes.

Q. Thank you, Dr. Annand! Now can I ask you, Dr. Annand, how do you fix the time that the operation lasted, at an hour and a half?

A. I said about an hour and a half. I give that time approximately.

Q. How many operations were performed that afternoon?

A. Two.

Q. Did the other operation precede this one?

A. Yes.

Q. What operation was it?

A. It commenced as an excision of the knee joint and ended in amputation through the thigh.

Q. By whom was that operation performed?

A. Mr. Beaney.

Q. Did he kill that man?

A. The patient was a woman and she is still alive.[2]

Q. How long did that operation take?

A. About an hour, but I did not time it.

Q. What time did the operations begin and at what time did they finish?

A. The first was commenced about three o'clock and the second one was finished at about half past five.

Q. Are you sure that the operation for amputation through the thigh did not take longer than an hour?

A. I am only saying what my opinion is; I did not time the operation.

---

2 See Epilogue for further information on this case.

Q. Do you know how long the administration of chloroform took for each patient?

A. I do not know.

Q. (moving to the table with the instruments) Now you say a suggestion was made to crush the stone?

A. Yes.

Q. Is the instrument here that was brought to Mr. Beaney during the operation?

A. It is here.

Q. (picking up one of the instruments and holding it towards the witness) Is this the one, the one with the key?

A. Yes I believe it is. All of the instruments were at hand in the instrument room, adjoining the operating theatre.

Q. How many were at hand?

A. The whole stock was in the adjoining room.

Q. Was any other lithotrite than this one brought?

A. There were three brought and all the lithotrites were available.

Q. But this is the one that was handed to Mr. Beaney?

A. Yes.

Q. Do you mean to say that this toy (holding the instrument high for everyone to see), this toy of a thing is applicable for crushing a calculus of large size in the bladder?

A. You can never tell until you make the attempt.

Q. Have you heard of the celebrated French operator Civiale?

A. I have heard of him.

Q. Well, Civiale describes an instrument, which looks like an ordinary lithotomy forceps but has a screw drill running down the centre and that screw engages the stone. [Jean Civiale first used this instrument, which he called his "trilabrium", successfully in Paris in 1824. It was later popularised in England by Henry Thompson.][3]

---

3 It was Thompson who was about to operate for a third time for stone on Napoleon III when the latter died and

(turning back to the witness) Now is there any such crushing instrument as that in the Melbourne Hospital?

A. No, not that I know of, but I do not have charge of the instruments.

Q. Did Mr. Beaney succeed in drawing the stone up to the mouth of the wound and did it not then slip back on more than one occasion?

A. Yes, he never could get it right out.

Q. Was it after the stone had constantly slipped that the scoop was used?

A. Yes.

Q. Did Dr. Beaney succeed in crushing a portion of the stone with the forceps?

A. A portion of the soft outside.

Q. He succeeded in breaking it off?

A. A great deal of debris came away.

---

was found to have his kidneys virtually destroyed by chronic infection.

Q. Dr. Annand, you are saying that he crushed it with the forceps to a certain extent?

A. Yes Mr. Beaney did attempt to crush the stone and did so to a certain extent.

Q. (allowing this response to settle with the jury) Dr. Annand do you recognise it as a fact that in practical surgery uncommon incidents may arise in the course of an operation, which may render it necessary to act on the spur of the moment, using one's best judgement?

A. Certainly that is the case.

Q. You will not attempt to deny that Mr. Beaney, as a rule, uses his best endeavours to show off his skill and that he is a man of considerable ability as a surgeon?

A. (swallowing, and turning to the Coroner) I don't know whether I should express an opinion about his ability, I don't think it is a fair question. If you think I should answer the question I will answer it.

The Coroner intervened, 'I do not believe it is appropriate for a junior doctor to comment on the capabilities of his seniors.'

Q. Very well. Dr. Annand, let us go back to the days before the operation. Were you present with Mr. Beaney in the dead house on the day preceding the operation?

A. I cannot say whether it was on the day preceding but I was there shortly before the operation.

Q. Who else was there?

A. There were some students.

Q. And did you see Mr. Beaney do anything there?

A. Yes, he practiced some operation on a dead body.

Q. What operation?

A. An operation for stone.

Q. Mr. Beaney rehearsed the operation of lithotomy on a dead subject before the operation?

A. Yes.

Q. How many bodies did he practice on?

A. Two.

Q. Did he not try on one body the median operation and on the other body the lateral operation to determine the space available?

A. Yes.

Q. You agree he operated on the two bodies to test the amount of space obtained by different operations?

A. Yes.

Q. There is no rule in the hospital rendering it imperative for an honorary surgeon to rehearse an operation before he performs it?

A. No.

Q. So that Mr. Beaney made this special effort in the interests of the patient, Robert Berth, upon whom he intended to operate the next day?

A. Yes.

Q. (pausing to let the response sink in, then returning to the instrument table to point to the two scoops) Are these two instruments the same as they were when the operation was completed?

A. No they have been straightened out since.

Q. Both of them?

A. One of them was bent and the spring of the other was broken.

Q. Who was using the one that was bent?

A. Mr. Webb and Mr. Beaney were both using the instruments but I cannot say who held the one that was bent.

Q. Dr. Annand, can we move on now to the stage after surgery. Prior to this man's death, was he not in a state of collapse?

A. The patient was in a state of collapse for about seven or eight hours before he died. He was given stimulants and calomel and port wine, as ordered by Mr. Beaney, as well as poultices to his wound.

Q. Do you know if this unfortunate man ever suffered from disease of urinary parts other than the kidney?

A. He had suffered from a discharge of mucus and bloody matter from the penis for some time.

Q. Would not that show organic disease, perhaps of the bladder?

A. Yes, it might.

With that Purves turned to the Coroner to indicate that he had no further questions of that witness.

The next witness called was Dr. John Williams, a resident physician at the Melbourne Hospital. He was a tall man, older than the usual resident by approximately a decade and indeed was about the same age as Purves. He had graduated in Edinburgh and practiced medicine in both England and the United States. He was in Chicago when Mary O'Leary's cow tripped over a lantern in the shed and started the great fire of 1871. He subsequently moved to Australia for his health as he had a respiratory complaint, which was greatly affected by the severe northern winters. Nevertheless he was known to be a hard worker and was considered to have a good future in medicine. He was later to be recognised by students and residents as a superlative clinical teacher, and would in fact become the physician Beaney turned to in his final illness.

The Coroner established through some preliminary questions that Dr. Williams was indeed a resident physician of the hospital and had been among those present at the operation, but had not assisted. The Coroner then asked the witness to describe the operation as he saw it. Dr. Williams went on to outline how Mr. Beaney, seated in front of the patient's buttocks, made the initial incision and then in a 'hacking' manner cut down upon the metallic speculum that had been introduced into the anus.

Again Mr. Beaney rose to rebuke the witness for that description of his actions, shouting 'Nonsense!', which caused the witness to halt in mid-speech.

The Coroner turned to Mr. Beaney and advised him that this was his final warning not to interrupt. Mr. Beaney sat down without uttering another word, but glowered at the witness.

Dr. Williams continued, but being aware of Beaney's threatening countenance, stated that he was unsure of the exact details of the surgery. However he went on to describe how the stone was found to be larger than was thought and could not be drawn out by forceps. He indicated that scoops were then used and in the process one of the scoops was bent and the spring of the other was broken. He felt that a very great force had been used before the stone was finally levered out. He admitted that he had never seen a stone removed in that way before, nor had he heard of it being done. He thought he did hear someone suggest that the stone should be crushed but Dr. Beaney had remarked that he would like to get it out whole. He also indicated that he heard Dr. Annand mention the suprapubic operation and remembered Mr. Webb offering Mr. Beaney a lithotrite, but smaller he recalled than the one that had been produced at the inquest. In concluding his responses to the

Coroner's questions, he thought that the operation had taken an hour and a half.

Mr. Purves then moved to cross-examine him, asking him first if he was a surgeon. To Mr. Purves's surprise the witness responded that he was. To Dr. Williams MB (Bachelor of Medicine) meant physician and surgeon, when he wished it to be so. Melbourne University at that time only awarded an MB, not the MBBS (Bachelor of Medicine. Bachelor of Surgery) it later awarded,[4] and it became quite a problem in hospital appointments for new graduates wishing to follow a surgical career.

Q. Have you done this operation yourself?

A. I have never performed it myself.

Q. Have you seen it performed?

A. I have seen it done.

Q. How many times?

A. I could not tell you.

Q. Do you know what Lloyd's operation is?

---

4 The medical course at Melbourne University is now a four-year postgraduate course, with the degree of Doctor of Medicine (MD) being awarded.

A. I am not sure.

Purves then held up the speculum that had been used at the operation.

Q. What is the slit in this instrument for?

A. I imagine it is made with the intention that it should be cut into.

Q. Dr. Williams, in responding to the Coroner's question you said that there was no cut into the rectum with a knife. Now as a surgeon you would therefore know this. You know that this particular instrument is used to guide the scalpel of the operator when cutting into the rectum. Would a surgeon introduce a speculum except for that reason?

A. I have not the least idea why it was introduced.

Q. (looking to the jury in mock bewilderment) Do you still say there was no cut in the rectum?

A. There was not.

Q. If another witness swore differently would you venture to contradict him?

A. Yes, I think I could.

Purves almost slammed the speculum down on the instrument table with a very deliberate movement, the noise of it hitting the table reverberating in the courtroom. He then held up a forceps and turned back to the witness, and asked him if he agreed from the position the handles were in that the stone must have been a large one. The witness agreed that it was most likely a large stone, but could not recall whether or not Mr. Beaney had said at the operation that it was large.

Q. When removal of the stone was not successful with the forceps were scoops used?

A. Yes.

Q. Was one scoop introduced under the object and the other placed over it?

A. Yes, that was the way.

Q. And force was then used to bear down on the top scoop in order to press it against the lower scoop?

A. Yes.

Q. Was Mr. Beaney holding one scoop and Mr. Webb holding the other one?

A. Yes.

Q. Do you recall whether it was the scoop held by Mr. Beaney orthe one held by Mr. Webb that was bent?

A. They were both bent.

Q. (holding up one of the scoops) Is not this one of the scoops actually used?

A. I do not know.

Q. (moving closer to the witness and bending one of the scoops) Is that a fair example of the instruments used at the hospital? Is that the sort of thing a man's life aught to depend upon?

A. It all depends upon how the instrument is used.

Q. (picking up the scoop with the spring mechanism) Is this the same spring scoop that was used?

A. Yes, I believe so.

Q. And do you see here that the spring is broken? Do you call that a powerful instrument?

A. It is, for the purpose for which it was made; it is a powerful instrument for traction.

Q. (slowly) Instrument for traction ... You heard Dr. Annand suggest the suprapubic operation to remove the stone?

A. Yes.

Q. Would you venture to say that with an empty bladder that would be a safe operation to undertake?

A. Undoubtedly an empty bladder would be disadvantageous.

Q. Could it be attempted, without facing some great and inevitable danger?

A. No, it could not.

Q. That danger is injury to the peritoneum resulting in peritonitis?

A. Yes.

Q. Would you, knowing that the bladder could not be distended, still cut into the patient's belly to get the stone out that way?

A. I would take the matter into serious consideration.

Q. Knowing that the bladder was empty?

A. (hesitating, sweat appearing on his forehead) Knowing that the bladder was empty I still might consider doing so. I think it might be possible to push the peritoneum aside.

Q. But don't you have to cut down on it in order to be able to push it aside and you would have no staff to guide the blade of the sharp instrument?

A. The operation would then become more difficult but it still might be possible.

Q. Possible but not probable. (pausing) If you failed with the suprapubic operation would you adopt the lateral?

A. No, I would not for I would know that I must succeed.

Q. In killing the patient?

A. In getting out the stone.

Q. (picking up an instrument from the table for the witness to see) The only lithotrites in the hospital are similar in formation to this one?

A. I believe so.

Q. And one similar to this was brought to Mr. Beaney?

A. Yes.

Q. Do you, as a physician and a surgeon, believe that this lithotrite is capable of crushing that large stone?

A. I believe it would.

Q. Would you risk your life on such an instrument?

A. I do not think that is a question you should put. I am not in a position to require such an instrument.

Q. Would you back yourself against death that that particular instrument would crush that particular stone?

A. If I had the preference of having that stone crushed by that instrument or pulled out, I would have it crushed.

Q. That is no answer. You have had a week to think over the matter and have conversed on the subject with other medical men. Do you believe that the instrument that I have here would crush that large stone?

A. (with some hesitation) I think it would.

Q. (placing the instrument back on the table and returning to the witness) How did you come to meet with Dr. Barker and Dr. Neild privately at Dr. Barker's house?

A. Well some fluid was taken out of the pelvis and was put in to a soda water bottle and....

Q. Was it at your desire that the consultation took place or did they invite you?

A. No I was about to say I had taken notes at the post-mortem examination and....

Q. Did you all three put your heads together?

A. What do you mean?

Q. Did you consult together and reason out and discuss the case?

A. We certainly did.

Q. The other two gentlemen are your seniors are they not?

A. Yes they are.

Q. I suppose your mind yielded somewhat to their persuasive arguments?

A. There was no need for yielding.

Q. You were all of one mind?

A. Yes, pretty well so.

Q. Dr. Barker's ideas and your ideas coincided?

A. Certainly not in all things. If you mean that generally we came to the same conclusions, I say yes.

Q. Your sympathies were with Dr. Barker and Nield? I had no sympathies in the matter at all.

Q. Do know what a calculus is made of?

A. The centre of most is formed from uric acid and the outer part by phosphates.

Q. And is the centre very hard?

A. Yes.

Purves loudly repeated the words "very hard" and turning to the Coroner said that he had. no more questions of this witness.

Before the witness stepped down the Coroner asked some further questions.

Q. How long have you been in the hospital?

A. I only started there the day before I witnessed the operation. Before then I only knew the resident medical officers.

Q. Was it then that you first met Dr. Beaney?

A. Yes I was introduced to Mr. Beaney for the first time then.

Q. So that you had no prejudices at all events?

A. I had no prejudices on the subject then, nor have I now.

With some relief Dr. Williams then stepped down.

The next witness was Dr. John James Colquhoun Dempster. Dempster like the majority of doctors in the colony had been trained in the British Isles. He had settled in mid Victoria and had a large and busy practice, such that he generally needed more than one assistant doctor to help him with the workload. He entered the witness stand with a more confident manner than that which the previous witnesses had displayed. However, the conservative nature of his dress was quite the opposite of Beaney's and whilst the Coroner was swearing him in it is likely that Purves would have wondered which way his sympathies might fall.

The Coroner asked the witness if he was present at the operation and the witness confirmed that he had been present by invitation. The Coroner then asked him for a summary of the events of the operation.

> A. Dr. Beaney performed a modification of the median operation. He cut so as to reach the stone very well. It was at once evident that the stone was a very large one – exceptionally large. He attempted to extract it with the forceps several times, but the surface of the stone broke away on one or two occasions and caused his forceps to slip off. Eventually, Mr. Webb and he extracted it with the scoops. I think the operation took altogether about 40 minutes. In fact I am certain as to the time within a few minutes, because I looked at my watch. The whole operation took between 40 and 50 minutes from the administration of the chloroform to the end of the operation.
>
> Q. Was the stone levered out?

A. It was extracted by a combination of force and leverage with the two scoops. Mr. Beaney had his scoop underneath and Mr. Webb his scoop above, pressing on it so as to prevent hurting the soft parts. The stone required great force. It came out with a jump. It was more levered out than extracted. There was considerable force used but it was necessary, I suppose, to get it out. I judge that from the fact of the forceps slipping off the stone.

Pleased with this testimony, Mr. Purves moved to cross-examine.

Q. Were you with Mr. Beaney when he rehearsed the operation on a dead body previously?

A. No. I knew very little of Mr. Beaney.

Q. Have you seen any operations for the stone before?

A. I have seen lots of operations performed. I spent some years with Mr. Fergusson in England.

Q. Fergusson! You mean the great surgeon of King's College Hospital and Surgeon to the Queen.

A. Yes, I do mean him and I have seen the lateral and the median operations performed during my time in England.

The Coroner intervened, 'Have you ever seen a stone as large as this extracted?'

> A. No. I suggested to Mr. Beaney that he crush the stone, but I saw no instrument there suitable. These instruments (glancing at the instruments laid out on the table and scornfully gesturing to them) are powerless for such work. I looked over the table of instruments in the operating room but saw nothing fit to do it. There is a particular type of forceps made for crushing large stones, which can be introduced through the wound, but it was not present amongst them.

The Coroner responded. 'If you had been performing the operation would you have not seen that there was an instrument there with which to crush the stone if necessary?'

> A. I do not think that there is an instrument in Melbourne that could crush that particular stone!

Mr. Purves resumed questioning.

> Q. Can you ascertain the size of the stone beforehand?

> A. To a certain extent, but not to a nicety. A stone of that size would occupy a large amount of space in the bladder, making the manipulation of the forceps to measure the size of the stone

difficult. Mr. Beaney got the stone out of the bladder several times but it slipped back again.

Q. Did you see any neglect or want of care?

A. I saw a good deal of force used, but no neglect or want of care.

Q. There are many cases, I suppose both medical and surgical, where it becomes absolutely necessary for a medical man at some particular juncture to make up his mind at once and to act.

A. Of course.

Q. There was no instrument there to crush that stone?

A. No. There was not.

Q. (with emphasis) There was not. (turning to the Coroner). No further questions.

The Coroner however had some further questions.

Q. Was there nothing there at all with which he could have attempted to crush the stone?

A. The stone was of exceptional size, weighing 6 1/2oz, and would require a very powerful instrument. Mr. Beaney asked my opinion on the case and at his request I examined the man before the extraction of the stone.

Q. What would have you done had it been your case?

A. I would have divided the other side of the prostate gland. If I had had a proper instrument I would have crushed the stone.

Q. Would you have adopted the suprapubic operation?

A. I think not.

Q. Would not this lithotrite have been powerful enough to crush it?

A. I do not think there would have been sufficient room in the instrument to grasp it.

Q. Thank you. You are excused.

The last witness for the morning was Dr. Patrick Moloney. He was only 32 years of age and had been appointed as an honorary physician to the Melbourne Hospital earlier in the year when Beaney was re-elected. He was a first generation Australian of Irish parents and was one of only three students enrolled in the new medical course at the Melbourne

University in 1862. He became a resident physician at the Melbourne Hospital in 1867 and worked hard over the long hours of that demanding position. Being a quick-tempered young man, on more than one occasion during his term as a resident he fought with the authorities to obtain a little more leave than was traditionally granted to the residents. However, overall he was popular and he was competent. When he later applied for a senior appointment the hospital felt that it would benefit from having the first Australian medical graduate on the staff. He was original in his thinking and whilst this did not make him a good teacher of students, who needed (or thought they did) didactic instruction, he was a welcome and innovative educator of those residents, who later were to work with him. For example, believing they would be effective, he prescribed marrowbones (as they contained red cells) for anaemic young women. He also recognised the need to correct the debilitating dehydration of typhoid fever patients, although he had no effective way at that time of correcting their fluid and electrolyte losses, as systems for intravenous infusion had not been developed.

Like many an Irishman he had a fondness for alcohol, which he regarded as an excellent travelling companion. He also wrote poetry and was an admirer of literary men of the day such as Marcus Clarke, Adam Lindsay Gordon and Henry Kendall, who met regularly at the Yorick Club.

The Coroner established that Dr. Moloney was an honorary physician to the Melbourne Hospital and was present at the operation, but not at its commencement.

Q. Was the bladder cut into when you got there?

A. Yes.

Q. The principal part of the operation was done by that time?

A. Yes.

Q. Describe what you saw.

A. The first thing I saw was that Mr. Beaney had hold of a very large stone with a pair of forceps. He had pulled the stone several times to the mouth of the external wound and in the process some outside pieces of the stone chipped off. I saw Mr. Webb assisting him by using a scoop, placing it behind the stone. Together they levered it out with considerable force.

Q. Was there, do you think, sufficient force to seriously injure the soft parts at the time and cause the man to suffer from such a severe operation itself, where the body parts were so much dilated?

A. I do not think that more force was used than was necessary

Q. Was the force used sufficient to injure the soft parts?

A. Yes.

Q. What else do you recall of the operation?

A. When Mr. Beaney remarked to me that it was an unusually large stone, having seen the stone got so close to the outside, I asked "Cannot you crush it", or something to that effect. I turned to the lithotomy instruments and selected the largest one I could find.[5]

Q. You selected the largest instrument?

A. Yes.

Q. Did you hand it to him?

A. Mr. Beaney inspected the instrument, but as he looked at it I made the remark that I did not think it was strong enough for the purpose. Mr.

5 Such was the lack of awareness of the need for sterility that even an observer could handle the operating instruments.

Webb, I think, then took the instrument in his hand and put it down near Mr. Beaney but I do not think it was used.

Mr. Purves was then invited to cross-examine the witness.

Q. You say that Mr. Beaney did not use the instrument you had held up.

A. No, I do not think so.

Q. You know that there are improvements being made in surgical instruments every day?

A. Yes.

Q. You won't attempt to say that these ones displayed (gesturing at the instruments) are the latest and the best inventions for crushing stone in the bladder?

A. No, but there are other lithotrites than those you produced.

Q. You have been some years in the Melbourne Hospital have you not?

A. Yes, if you include my resident years.

Q. Do you know how often this stock of instruments has been renewed?

A. No, I cannot say.

Q. Would you consider that if any instrument bends, in the way the one produced has, then it would be a proper one to use?

A. I have seen instruments bend and break in operations, but that is not a usual thing.

Purves indicated that he had no further questions of the witness. The Coroner however had some.

Q. What would you have done under the circumstance you have described?

A. There are two courses open, either to enlarge the opening of the wound or decrease the size of the stone.

Q. What would you have done?

A. Under the circumstances the stone could not be crushed. If the lithotrite had broken in the bladder it might have left a part there and that would have increased the injuries. That lithotrite I was shown would have had no effect upon the stone at all; it would just lift it up and no more.

Q. Do you think it would have been safer to have enlarged the wound or broken the stone?

A. There is a difference of opinion among surgeons as to whether it was better, when the stone was found to be larger than expected, to dilate the wound or to enlarge it by cutting. The modern tendency on this vexed question is I think in favour of cutting. The chipping away of portions of the outside of the stone indicated that it was softer in some parts than others. If the whole stone had been phosphate it could easily have been crushed.

From his chair Purves was heard again to repeat 'There is a difference of opinion amongst surgeons' before some words of his own, 'as to what to do in such a circumstance.'

The inquest was adjourned for lunch.

Purves, Duffett and Beaney had a brief luncheon at a nearby hotel on the northwest corner of Swanston and Flinders Streets, a favourite drinking spot for Melbourne's young rowers at that time. It must have been difficult however to have a conversation, with noisy interruptions coming not so much from the bar trade as from the sounds of builders working. The new owners Young and Jackson, two young miners who had made their fortune in New Zealand, had commenced renovations after buying the hotel just a few months before. Thus Beaney did not hear all of the exchanges between his defending barrister and solicitor but did catch an odd sentence or two, one of which was the mention of Rule 7, concerning consultations. Although Beaney didn't think it of importance, Duffett saw it as one of the major points against his client.

Purves was reasonably confident that there had been no damning evidence from the resident staff and that on the other hand Dempster and Moloney have been of considerable value to their case. Both Purves and Duffett doubted whether the Coroner would have established the inquest on the basis of the evidence available so far. Both agreed there must be something else that influenced the Coroner, something that was yet to come out. Perhaps the key lay with Webb, who, in assisting Beaney, would have had the closest opportunity to observe Beaney's performance.

Had Beaney made some other serious error of judgement, which had not yet come to light? Would another surgeon, such as the eminent Thomas Fitzgerald, have done something different and the patient survived. This was not a question that either lawyer felt they could put to Beaney, but given Dempster's evidence it was in any case unlikely.

Purves had never met Thomas Fitzgerald, who was also on the honorary medical staff at the Melbourne Hospital, but had been in his house, Rostella, a most handsome Regency building, which was in Lonsdale Street close to Williams Street. During the building of the Supreme Court, Fitzgerald had allowed the large ballroom of his house to be used as a court for civil cases and Purves had appeared there. He remembered, amongst the paintings on the wall, one titled *Chloé* by Jules Lefebvre. It was of a young nude woman standing erect, a striking picture. It was painted in the 1870s and it had won for Lefebvré the grand medal of honour at the Paris Salon. Fitzgerald had paid 850 guineas for it. A guinea, being one pound and one shilling, was an amount commonly used in professional fees, a hangover from a guinea coin, which was popular in England in the 18th century. Purves could not know that the painting would prove an embarrassment to Fitzgerald in later years when he lent it to the National Gallery. As the gallery was open on Sundays it led to the trustees being attacked by the Presbyterian Assembly, for displaying such a painting on the Sabbath. Argument for and against took place in the columns of the *Argus* for a month but eventually it was withdrawn. Purves also could not have known that on Fitzgerald's death Young and Jackson would purchase that same painting for £800, and hang it in the very place where they were then meeting. It would be over a century before the beautiful but bare Chloe would win back respectability and once more hang in the gallery, albeit for a short time only, while Young and Jackson's was again undergoing renovations. There was no commotion over her second coming to the gallery. The Rev. Strong's early addresses had not all been in vain. The real life Chloé was a model of Persian descent. Her name was

Marie and she was nineteen at the time of the painting. Sadly she suicided a few years later, the rumour being that it was because of her unrequited love for Lefebvré.

8. Webb weaving

The first witness called, following the midday break, was Mr. John Holden Webb M.R.C.S. Webb was thirty-five and, as mentioned earlier, had been appointed an assistant surgeon to the Melbourne Hospital when Beaney was re-appointed. He was South African born but studied in England and took his medical training at St. Mary's Hospital. When he came to Australia, not long after graduating, he obtained a resident surgeon post at the Amherst Hospital before starting up private surgical practice in Melbourne. The town of Amherst grew on the site of one of the richest goldfields discovered in mid-Victoria in 1853. Most of the township would in later years be destroyed by a bushfire, and little of it remains other than the Amherst cemetery. Some eccentricities about Webb were his rapid speech, making him at times a little difficult to understand, and the overuse of his hands in gesticulating whilst speaking, somewhat like a comic might do in later years in the silent movies of the early1900s.

The Coroner established Mr. Webb's qualifications and his appointment as an assistant honorary surgeon at the Melbourne Hospital and then asked him if he had been acquainted with the deceased, Robert Berth.

> A. Yes, I received a note from a medical man in the town of Talbot stating that he had a case of

stone in the nearby Amherst Hospital and asked me if I would like to get the man a bed in the Melbourne Hospital and operate on him myself. We had had several cases of stone together before that, two or three. He told me the stone was fairly large and I mentioned the case to Mr. Beaney, who said he did not think the committee would like me to operate myself. Berth came down to my place at East Melbourne and on the day following, whilst there, was taken very ill from the exertions consequent upon the long journey down to Melbourne. While Berth was at my house he was so ill that he lay on my couch for several hours. He took lodgings in a neighbouring hotel until I could get him a bed at the hospital.

Q. Did you see him at the hospital?

A. I saw him.

Q. Did you mention to Mr. Beaney the state the man was in?

A. I told him he was not a strong man.

Q. Did you tell him of the illness he had suffered from whilst in your house?

A. No, I did not think of it at the time.

Q. You were present at the operation?

A. I was and I assisted.

Q. Tell me what you saw.

A. Mr. Beaney had got hold of the stone between the forceps and worked it from side to side for the purpose of dilating the wound with forceps. The stone slipped away from the forceps in the most provoking way. Mr. Beaney afterwards caught the stone by its long diameter and exclaimed (throwing up his arms as he continued) My God! What a large stone it is. I then said to him "What do you think of crushing it?" For a few minutes Mr. Beaney was dilating with his thumb and finger until he could get hold of the stone. During this time part of it broke off, and when it appeared to be almost extracted it slipped back again. It was most aggravating. Mr. Beaney said to me-"See if you can get hold of it" and just then it slipped back a third time. I then took up the lithotrite and said to Mr. Beaney "What do you think of that?" He looked at the instrument but was disdainful of it so I put it down again. Then Mr. Beaney said to me "See if you cannot hold it." One of the students then handed me another instrument (pointing to a particular lithotrite on the table, after which the clerk brought it to him). And I said, "I am afraid this will break, this sort of thing is of no use."

Webb began opening and closing the instrument as he spoke, and then the instrument broke.

Mr. Purves was on his feet in an instant and said to the jury 'You see gentlemen the instrument has just broken whilst in use.'

The witness then continued.

> A. The lithotrite worked more easily than it did just now but it was really no good at all. Mr. Beaney turned around to the gentlemen present at the operation and said "Well it is almost impossible to get out." I said, "It is caught under the pubic symphysis." Mr. Beaney then passed a scoop up under the stone and said "I think I can do it now." I got another scoop and put it on the stone but I found that I needed to go around to the other side of the patient to apply some pressure. In doing so I pressed with the scoop on the upper part of the stone, down towards the bottom scoop. The stone then rolled out between the two scoops and fell on to the ground.

The Coroner went on.

> Q. Did you bend the scoop in doing so?

> A. Certainly I did.

> Q. This scoop is not intended to be used with force?

A. A fair amount of force is always allowed in a case like this.

Q. You were using one kind of instrument and put that down to take another?

A. Sometimes when you cannot get the instrument you want you must take what you can get.

A juryman, Frederick Fanning, who was a skilled tradesman, then intervened with a question directly to the witness.

Q. Have you had any experience in operating for stone?

A. I was house surgeon to the Lock Hospital in London and the nearby St. Peter's Hospital, a special one for stone. [6] In St. Peter's Hospital there are more operations performed than in any two hospitals in the United Kingdom, excepting for the Norwich Hospital.[7] I have seen, I believe, more than 100 operations for stone.

---

6 The Lock Hospital was originally established for the treatment of venereal diseases. Both it and St Peters hospitals continued to function until the middle of the 20th century.

7 The large Norwich Hospital in Norfolk functioned until 2003.

The Coroner continued.

Q. Have you ever seen a stone got out in this way before?

A. No, I never did, but I never saw so large a stone. (using both hands, in a slightly exaggerated manner, he indicated a mass larger than a cricket ball)

Getting to his feet, Mr. Purves said: "I never saw so large a stone." He then commenced the cross-examination.

Q. During an operation at any time when a stone appears to be almost extracted is it a common thing to use forceps for dilation?

A. Yes.

Q. To dilate the prostate gland, which I understand is about the size of a walnut?

A. Yes.

Q. Do you believe along with Erichsen, in spite of Dr. Barker, that dilatation means laceration?

A. I certainly do.

Here the Coroner intervened.

Q. Are you saying that when you operate on the prostate gland you must always lacerate?

A. Yes.

Mr. Purves resumed.

Q. When the pressure was brought to bear on the scoop you used, the force would act upon the side of the stone and upon the bottom scoop held by Mr. Beaney?

A. Yes, then the stone rolled out. If I knew all about the stone then, as I do now, I could take it away as easily as possible.

With that reply the witness had stretched out his hand in front of him and drew it back, slowly making some rotating movements with the hand. Purves quickly moved on.

Q. You have read from what disease the late Emperor Napoleon suffered?

A. Yes.

Q. Do you know what the disease known as surgical kidney is?

A. Yes, I know the disease. The Emperor Napoleon died from acute pyelitis, from the pressure of the stone upon the orifice of the bladder, impeding the flow of water.

Q. That would cause inflammation?

A. Yes; it is a disease that often slumbers for years and then lights up after some interference with the genital organs. One kidney alone is usually affected and those organs are discovered to be enlarged and engorged with blood.

The Coroner interspersed:

Q. Then this disease does not show itself during life?

A. No. The authorities say that you cannot tell of its existence. Certainly in the Emperor's case the disease was not suspected.

Purves went on.

Q. How long did the operation on Berth last?

A. I cannot tell, there were so many things passing before me.

Purves then indicated that he had no further questions. The Coroner however, did have some.

Q. (leaning toward the witness) Would you have used the lithotrite, Mr. Webb?

A. I think I would but it is a very difficult instrument to use.

Q. Is it not an operation that is very often performed? I am aware that the English surgeon, Sir Henry Thompson, did not take long to collect the materials for publishing 200 cases.

A. That is true, but Sir Henry Thompson had cases of stone coming to him, at the University Hospital London, from all parts of the world.

The Coroner gazed at the witness for around half a minute as if he wished to ask further questions, but then advised the witness that he could stand down but that he might be recalled later in the inquiry.

The next witness was Mr. James Williams, who had been Secretary of the Melbourne Hospital for twenty-one years. He was a competent accountant and successful fundraiser, having played a large role in the founding of Hospital Sunday. He was not particularly popular with the nursing staff, however, nor with the honorary medical staff, some of whom he handled with difficulty. He was more than a little in awe of James Beaney, whose disposition he had disturbed on several occasions over the alcohol issue.

Unlike the hospitals of today there was no sizeable management structure, no profession of health care administrators. Hospitals were run by a Board, generally on the advice of its medical staff, and to a greater or lesser extent the matron (in charge of nursing). Williams held the position of Hospital Secretary for such a long period not only through his competency but because, having little executive power, he represented no challenge to any of the senior people at the hospital. The Coroner established that he was the secretary of the hospital and then asked him if he could produce the rules of the Melbourne Hospital. Williams replied in the affirmative, stating in doing so that they were framed by the committee under the Parliament's *Hospital Act.*

The Coroner asked if all of the medical officers of the institution had been sent a copy of the rules and if, in particular, a copy had been sent to Mr. Beaney on his reappointment to the hospital. Mr. Williams replied that Mr. Beaney had been sent a copy of the rules.

The Coroner then asked the witness what the rules were with reference to operations and he responded that operations were dealt with under Rule 7.

With that the witness handed a copy of the rules to the Coroner at which point the Coroner turned to the jury and said, 'Gentlemen this is Rule Number 7':

> No important operation in surgery shall be performed without the previous consent of the patient (if in a position to give it), nor unless sanctioned on a consultation by two at least of the surgeons, except in the case of an emergency. All consultations (cases of emergency excepted) shall be held on Tuesday in the consultation room.

> The result of each consultation shall be entered in the consultation book, to which the surgeons present shall attach their signatures. All capital operations (cases of emergency excepted) shall be performed at two o'clock on Mondays and Thursdays. Unless absolutely necessary, no operation shall be performed on Sunday.

The Coroner added, 'by way of explanation, gentlemen, a capital operation is one involving risk to life, and the operation undergone by this patient would fall into that category'. He then dismissed the witness but retained the written copy of the rule. Purves made no attempt to challenge him on the question of the gravity of the stone operation.

The next witness was Dr. Augustus Lewellin, a resident physician at the Melbourne Hospital. Lewellin had graduated from Melbourne University in 1872. The degree awarded by the University was M.B. only (as noted earlier) and Lewellin had just recently applied to transfer from house physician across to the surgical side. As the hospital bylaws recognised surgical qualifications only from the Royal Colleges in the United Kingdom, his transfer was refused and it took many months to resolve the problem. In the meantime Lewellin stayed with the administration of anaesthetics and he continued in this discipline, even when later he obtained the post of Medical Superintendent in the 1880s.

The Coroner established that Lewellin was a resident physician at the Melbourne Hospital, that he had administered chloroform to the patient Berth on December 2nd. The Coroner then questioned the witness further.

Q. How long did the operation last?

A. The patient was under chloroform only an hour and a half.

Q. How did you estimate the time?

A. I looked at my watch before the operation was commenced and after it was over.

Q. Did you see the operation at all or were you attending to the chloroform?

A. I saw a portion of the operation once or twice.

Q. Did you hear any proposition made to crush the stone?

A. I heard Mr. Webb propose to crush the stone.

Q. What did Mr. Beaney say?

A. He said "No! I would like to get it out whole."

Q. Did you see any force used in extracting the stone?

A. I saw Mr. Beaney one time use force with the forceps – considerable force.

Q. With the forceps?

A. Yes.

Q. You did not see the levers used at all?

A. No.

Q. Did Mr. Beaney say the stone was a large one or a small one?

A. Before he commenced to operate he said "As the stone is a small one I shall do the median operation".

Lewellin was then cross-examined by Mr. Purves, who had only two questions.

Q. I suppose you were wholly engaged in attending to your particular duty?

A. Yes.

Q. And your whole attention should be devoted to your duty of chloroform administration?

A. Yes.

Dr. Lewellin stood down, obviously relieved at the brief and stress-free examination he had undergone.

The next witness was a Dr. William Stewart Smythe, a practitioner from Sandridge (now Port Melbourne). Although in general practice, Smythe had gathered considerable minor surgical experience through the repair of wounds resulting from the many violent infractions, which occurred in that neighbourhood, particularly amongst its itinerant seafaring population. He had been in court just a few months before, giving evidence on a case in which the owner of the local Army and Navy Hotel, a retired sea captain called Harry Hall, was accused of biting off another man's nose. The hotel, in Dow Street, was opposite a large hall where the members of the various military brigades (drawn up in fear of that Russian invasion threat) practiced their drilling, after which their thirsts were quenched and arguments settled across the road at the Army and Navy Hotel. The original building, constructed in 1866, still stands but it is no longer a hotel.

It was established that Dr. Smythe had received an invitation from Mr. Beaney to attend the operation but as he sat in the amphitheatre he heard none of the conversation. He did contribute however that he thought the operation took about one hour, including the administration of chloroform and that the stone had been reached and seized in what he considered a very reasonable time, judging from his experience of over 50 operations for stone in both England and America. Purves did not ask any questions of Smythe but during Smythe's evidence Purves provoked the Coroner twice. The first time he accused the Coroner that when he demonstrated an instrument to a witness he invariably chose the wrong one, and the second time he accused the Coroner of putting questions that had been suggested by the detectives. The Coroner objected particularly to this latter accusation and indicated that he was in a two-fold position, having to be Prosecutor and Judge and he felt that he was exercising a very fair discretion. In response Purves muttered 'Much better than usual.'

Others who gave evidence during that long and hot afternoon were Dr. Edward Heffernan, a young graduate, who was present at the operation only for a short time and contributed little in the way of extra information; Dr. James Campbell Duncan, the resident surgeon who was in charge of the instruments, and claimed that he had crushed a piece of road metal three quarters of an inch thick with one of the hospital lithotrites; and Mr. John Jones, the surgical instrument maker who, in answer to a question from the Coroner, indicated that it would require a force of about 25 pounds to bend the scoops which had been used.

The Coroner then indicated that he would draw proceedings for the day to a close. He also advised that he wished to recall Mr. Webb, stating that he found the statement Webb had given to the police was quite at variance with evidence he had given during the inquest and this warranted a further explanation. Mr. Webb, still in the court, stood up and called out "How at variance?"

It is likely that at this point Purves realised that he was right and that the decision to hold the inquest lay with Webb's statement. He felt that it might be wise to try to assist Webb in avoiding the recall. He stood up, turned to Webb and stated, "You are entitled to know all the circumstances connected with a re-examination and you can only be recalled by the express permission of the Coroner."

The Coroner intervened, 'I do wish to recall him but in the first place I shall ask Detective Duncan to read the statement which Webb made to him.'

Purves, still on his feet, asked, 'Is this gentleman, on the mere statement of a detective, to be tried by this jury for perjury?'

'I am not going to charge him with perjury,' replied the Coroner, 'but I think he should give an explanation of his evidence, because it was upon his statement and similar statements that the body of the deceased was exhumed and all this inquiry and trouble were brought about.'

'I have serious doubts,' said Purves, 'as to whether this inquiry was brought about by any statement made by Mr. Webb and when I address the jury I will point out how, in my opinion, it arose.'

'We will take Detective Duncan's evidence first up tomorrow.' said the Coroner. 'Be careful, Mr. Purves, as I indicated earlier you will be allowed plenty of time to provide your opinion. This is not the Bloody Assizes of 1685. Unlike Baron Jeffreys who presided there and Mr. Beaney's late patient, I do not have a bladder stone that would force me to curtail proceedings.'

Apparently Judge Jeffreys speedily sentenced 331 Monmouth rebels to death during the trial, without allowing any arguments of self-defence, as he had to empty his irritated bladder hourly.

The following day was much cooler, which suited all concerned but particularly Purves who had not wished to make a summation to a hot, tired and sleepy jury, as they had seemed to him to be, at the end of the previous day's proceedings. He wanted their full attention when the time came.

As arranged, Detective Duncan was questioned first by the Coroner. John Duncan was quite experienced in giving evidence as he had had many court experiences and would have more in the years to come, including one in which he himself was the defendant in a trial in the Echuca Court, charged with cruelty to a prisoner. He was up there in the Murray River town tasked with transporting a prisoner between gaols, when the prisoner escaped. Duncan was said to have assaulted and kicked the prisoner at his recapture. Fortunately for Duncan the prisoner retracted much of his statement in the proceedings and Duncan was exonerated.

Duncan clarified the circumstances of his involvement in the Berth case in the typical constabulary monotone thought necessary for displaying disinterest or lack of bias and for dealing with the facts only.

The Coroner then proceeded to question him.

> Q. Did you see Mr. Webb about this subject?
>
> A. I did, but not first. I called on several medical men before seeing Mr. Webb. From the gentlemen I first called upon I received certain particulars in connection with the case and when I saw Mr. Webb, I read him the particulars I obtained. I have those particulars in my hand.
>
> Q. Will you read them?
>
> A. Yes. I said to Dr. Webb "Do you agree with what is mentioned here or do you differ from it?" He said: "I agree with it." I said: "Well now Dr. Webb will you be good enough to answer me a few questions?". He said: "I will." I said: "Did you take part in the operation?" He replied: "I did." I said: "To what extent?" He said: "I was there under Mr. Beaney assisting him, in the same position as a lieutenant under a captain. I was bound to do as I was told." I said: "Very good, doctor. Was there an incision made in the bladder

> for the purpose of inserting any instrument?" He said: "There was." I said: "Who made the incision?" He said: "Mr. Beaney." I said: "How was it made?" He said: "In a rather hacking sort of way."

A cry of denial came from Webb, who was sitting in the middle of the room. It was ignored by Detective Duncan, who continued with I said 'Go on, doctor.' He said: 'Forceps were inserted and the stone was caught hold of, then it slipped and part of the stone came away with the forceps.' I said, 'Was the stone what they call a phosphatic one?' He said, 'Yes.' He then went on to say Mr. Beaney made several efforts to remove the stone and failed and I then suggested to him to crush it. I then said: 'Now, doctor, supposing you had been the principal in this operation what mode would you have adopted?' and he said: "The suprapubic." I showed him this sketch (Duncan held up a sketch of the abdomen) and he pointed out the place in the lower part of a patient's abdomen, where the suprapubic operation should be effected. I then left his house and continued the inquiries elsewhere.'

Webb, jumped up and shouted at the witness: 'You say that I used the word hacking – I never used such a word.'

At this the Coroner intervened, 'Mr. Webb I shall call you shortly and take down any statement you wish to make, so please be seated and wait.'

Purves then cross-examined Duncan.

> Q. Who is the first medical man to whom you went and from whom you obtained a written report?
>
> A. I went to the hospital and saw Dr. Williams and Dr. Duncan together and Dr. Annand came in soon after.
>
> Q. I asked you who was the first one you saw?
>
> A. I saw both Dr. Duncan and Dr. Williams together.
>
> Q. You say you have a report in writing. From whom did you receive that?
>
> A. Dr. Williams. They were all together.
>
> Q. Who made the sketch?
>
> A. Dr. Duncan I think, but I am not sure.
>
> Q. Do you know who is the writer of the letter in the *Argus* signed A Practical Surgeon?
>
> A. I don't, I have not the remotest idea.

As Purves returned to his chair, the Coroner asked Mr. Webb if he wished to ask the witness any questions and Webb responded angrily 'I swear I never used the word hacking.'

Turning to Webb, Purves said 'I would certainly advise you not to ask a detective any more questions than you can help.'

Once Mr. Webb took the witness stand the Coroner asked him.

Q. What do you desire to state?

A. I did not use the word hacking. I said that the operation, so far as catching the stone, was done exceedingly well and I say so now.

Q. As regards the diagram or sketch?

A. I really do not know whether he showed it to me or not, I don't recollect it.

Q. Did you make any statement about the suprapubic operation?

A. No, I swear I did not. He may have used the word suprapubic and I had not listened to it. I am certain I did not use the word suprapubic to him. He may have asked me a question about it and I may have answered.

Q. Did you say it to anybody else?

> A. I may have done, I may have mentioned it at the time of the operation, I am not quite certain about that. I recall that I did say to Detective Duncan "Anything I have said you must not take as very material. For you to come here and me to answer your questions makes me look very much like a spy." (turning to the Coroner) There is just one other remark I wish to make. It has been reported that I stated that the patient suffered from the effects of the journey to Melbourne and that is true. He came to my house on the night of his arrival in Melbourne. I saw him next morning but not on the night of his arrival.

In dismissing the witness the Coroner said, 'If you want to correct all the little things in the newspapers to which you take exception your life will not be long enough for the task.'

Webb was shaking as he stood down. Whether it was from anger or fear for his future as a Melbourne Hospital surgeon one could not tell. He need not have worried. He later succeeded Girdlestone as the University lecturer in surgery and became recognised as an original and progressive surgeon. He had a strong interest in cancer and its causes and did some research in that field. In 1884 he wrote a seminal paper on the physical signs of acute appendicitis in which he described the site of maximum tenderness, which five years later was also described by the New

York surgeon Charles McBurney and was henceforth called McBurney's Point. It is known worldwide as such today by every student and surgeon, but it could have been Webb's Point.

The Coroner then addressed the jury. 'There are a number of other gentlemen here who were present at the operation. Are you satisfied with the evidence you have got or would you like any further evidence?'

Mr. Burton, the foreman, after consulting his brother jurymen replied: 'We have had quite enough.

Mr. Purves then stood up and said to the Coroner 'I suppose I may address a few remarks to the jury on the evidence?

'Yes,' the Coroner answered.

9. The plot won't succeed

Mr. Purves commenced his address. 'Gentlemen, you have already been, at considerable inconvenience to yourselves, engaged in a long and protracted inquiry as to the cause – the true and real cause – of the death of Robert Berth. No doubt, it is a most unfortunate thing that this poor creature, after years of suffering, should at last almost die upon the operating theatre table in the hospital. But that is by no means an uncommon fate with people who suffer from the dreadful disease known as a stone in the bladder. Fortunately, in recent years, through modern appliances, and especially from the use of chloroform and other anaesthetics, the pain of this terrible operation has been much diminished, and a new era in lithotomy has been established. Gentlemen, you must bear with me if I make any mistakes in the observations which I desire to address to you on this case, because up to the day before yesterday I really did not know what a lithotrite was, and knew very little about the operation of lithotomy. I shall, however, endeavour to put the case before you in plain English, because it seems to me that I ought to speak the language of common sense to men of common sense. Gentlemen, common sense will be your best guide throughout this inquiry; and doubtless you have paid every attention to all the evidence which has been placed before you.

'Now, it would be idle to deny – indeed, from the conduct of the examination by the learned professional gentleman who occupies the position of Coroner it is very evident – that the whole of this inquiry is directed against Dr. Beaney. In fact, you will be asked by the Coroner, who also acts as Crown Prosecutor in this case, if you think there is any evidence whatever to support this proceeding, to return a verdict that will be equivalent to a verdict of manslaughter against Dr. Beaney. You must not mince matters, that is the plain English of it; and that is why you have been brought here. The question is whether you are to return such a verdict.

'Gentlemen, I shall proceed to show you that there is not a tittle of evidence – not one single ground – for forever blasting the character of a man who, as a surgeon, holds a prominent position in this colony. Gentlemen don't let there be any accident with you. There may be accidents in the operating theatres of hospitals, but there should be no accident with you, who are capable of judging the evidence, which has been placed before you. And, before you begin to judge that evidence, I beg you – I most earnestly implore you – because it is my duty to do so, to reject all the statements with regard to this case, which you may have gathered from the daily prints.

'I say it with sorrow, that the newspaper, which purports to be the leading journal of this colony, has most indecently and most improperly alluded, not only to the facts of this case, which were known to the professional gentlemen who were involved, or who witnessed the operation, but also to the post-mortem examination, which was conducted within the building in which you are now sitting. Gentlemen, I say the evidence as it has come out here, as it has been elicited with great pains throughout the whole of this protracted inquiry, does not justify the biased paragraph which was printed and published before the inquest began.

'If the most diabolical enemy that Dr. Beaney has in the world, was to sit down, and, moved by malignant spite, was to attempt to describe the whole of the evidence which has been adduced, so as to make it appear in the most damaging way he could against that gentleman, I defy him to produce such a paragraph as the one which appeared in one of the morning newspapers before this inquest was commenced. That paragraph may have prejudiced your minds; you may have – in fact, I do not doubt that you did – come to this building with a foregone conclusion, in consequence of reading that paragraph. But I am happy to say that the responsibility, which rests on my shoulders, as counsel for Dr. Beaney, has been materially lessened. The responsibility, which I felt the day before yesterday, has been almost vanished away, by the evidence that has been given during the inquiry.

'Gentlemen, it is a singular fact that, in introducing the subject of the inquest to you, the Coroner was obliged to state that he was desirous to have the post-mortem examination of the body of the deceased performed by impartial persons. Whom did he succeed in getting to make the post-mortem examination? Dr. Barker, a rival of Dr. Beaney's, a gentleman who, no doubt would view an operation performed by his rival with suspicion, and who would be apt to judge harshly of any mistake made by Dr. Beaney, forgetting that he, perhaps, may have made mistakes in his time.

'Dr. Barker is one of the persons who made the postmortem examination, and who is the other? Dr. Neild, a literary and dramatic critic, a gentleman without any practice in his own profession, but with a knowledge of surgery which he refused to demonstrate to you in answer to the questions I put to him, and who exhibited a temper, which certainly was at variance with all my preconceived notions of what an impartial witness should be.

'You have to judge a witness by his demeanour, as well as by the language in which he couches his answer to the questions that are asked of him; and what was Dr. Neild's demeanour? The moment I asked him a question, it was like putting a spark into a powder barrel. He would not answer a single question, the reply to which would assist to enlighten you, as to the cause of the death of the unfortunate man Berth!.

'He knew all about the subject upon which I questioned him, but he would not communicate the knowledge which he possessed. He seemed to forget that he was here to inform you, to the upmost extent of his power, as to what was the cause of death.

'Gentlemen, I am here to help you arrive at a true and just conclusion on that point. My duty is not to endeavour to cast any distorting medium around the facts of this case, or any false glamour, but to assist you to judge the evidence fairly.

'What you have to decide is did Dr. Beaney, in the hospital, commit manslaughter, or murder? The two terms are almost synonymous. Now I will call your attention to two or three important passages, from a recognised legal authority, in regard to what amounts to manslaughter by a surgeon or physician. I quote from Russell on Grimes:

> And it seems now to be settled, that it makes no difference whether the party be a regular physician or surgeon or not. Thus it has been held, that if a person bona fide and honestly exercising his best skill to cure a patient, performs an operation, which causes the death of the patient, it makes no difference whether such person be a regular surgeon or not, nor whether he has had a regular education or not.
>
> A doctor was indicted for manslaughter, for causing death by thrusting a round piece of ivory against the rectum and thereby making a wound through the rectum for it appeared that, upon examination of the body after death, a small hole

> was discovered perforated through the rectum. The prisoner (the doctor) had attended the deceased, but there was no evidence to show how the wound had been caused, and questions were put in order to show that it might have been the result of natural causes. It was also proposed to show that the prisoner had had a regular medical education, and that a great number of cases had been successfully treated by him.

'In this case the judge, Baron John Hullock, stopping the case – as I imagined the Coroner would have stopped this inquiry yesterday – said

> This is an indictment for manslaughter, and I am really afraid to let the case go on, lest an idea should be entertained, that a man's practice may be questioned whenever an operation fails. In this case there is no evidence of the mode in which the operation was performed

'In the present case there is some evidence as to the mode in which the operation was performed; but in the case stopped by Baron Hullock there was no such evidence, and the learned judge went on to say

> Even assuming for the moment that it caused the death of the deceased, I am not aware of any law which says that this party can be found guilty of manslaughter. It is my opinion that it makes no difference whether the party be a regular or irregular surgeon.... It is quite clear that you may

> recover damages against a medical man for want of skill; but, as my Lord Hale,[8] says 'God forbid that any mischance of this kind should make a person guilty of murder or manslaughter.

'The authority from whom I am quoting adds

> Such is the opinion of one of the greatest judges that ever adorned the bench of the country. His proposition amounts to this, that if a person, bona fide and honestly exercising skill to cure a patient, performs an operation which causes the patient's death, he is not guilty of manslaughter.

'Well, gentlemen, you have to consider the question of how the operation in Berth's case was conducted. One point that is made against Dr. Beaney is that he ought to have known the precise size of the stone.

'Why, gentlemen, the text-books show that Erichsen, Civiale, Holmes, Cooper and Fergusson – I might go through the whole list of the great operators for stone – have all made mistakes. In fact, one man, as I read yesterday, made such mistakes in endeavouring to extract large stones that he set about and tried to invent an instrument for crushing stones in the bladder.

'How is it possible that any man, even if he introduced a lithotrite, which is suggested as the instrument with

---

8 Chief Justice of England in the 17th century.

which to measure a stone in the bladder, could ascertain the exact size of a stone? I say it is a physical and absolute impossibility for any man, be he a Barker, a Civiale, or a Cheselden, to measure the stone which was extracted from the deceased Berth with this instrument which only bites, when the first, second, third, or fourth screw of the worm has been introduced into the biting portion of the instrument.

'Suppose you are feeling, not in the light of day, but in a man's bladder – which is a dangerous operation even in itself, if the man has any predisposition towards disease – supposing you are feeling about in a man's bladder with an instrument of this kind, how can you tell the size of a stone in the bladder? How is it possible you can do that? You can judge it as a big one, no doubt, but it is impossible that you can judge its exact size, seeing that the gauge of the instrument is only scaled to 1 1/2 inches. Why, one of the chief causes of accident in connection with the operation of lithotomy, as laid down in Holmes's Surgery, from which I read a quotation yesterday, is the accidental discovery, during the operation, that the stone is of uncommon size.

'The stone, which was extracted in this case, is a stone of uncommon size. I suppose it is the largest stone, which was ever discovered in a man's bladder in so young a country as this. It is a stone of uncommon size, a rough stone, and one likely to injure the soft parts of the wound when being extracted.

'Now, gentlemen, Dr. Beaney did "sound" for stone, and it is said in the books that in sounding for stone great mistakes may be made. I read a list of cases of the kind to one of the witnesses, and I may repeat the substance from memory. Even Cheselden, the greatest operator who ever lived, operated three times for stone, and Samuel Cooper the great surgical writer and President of the College of Surgeons in London, seven times, and with what results in those cases? Why, having sounded for stone, having examined the bladder in every part, not only with a lithotrite but also with a sound, which is a thin narrow instrument – having adopted all these precautions – what did they do? Why, the patients were trussed up on the operating table, the operation was performed, and it was found that there was no stone in the bladder in any of these cases.

'Was there, however, any pretence whatever for saying that either of these great surgeons was guilty of manslaughter, because he made such a terrible mistake as that? The only mistake that Dr. Beaney can be said to have possibly made with regard to the stone in this case is that he thought it was smaller than it proved to be.

'Two or three witnesses have stated that Dr. Beaney said it was a small stone, and therefore he would do the median operation. Now, how can that be? Just let us look at the probabilities of the thing. Dr. Webb has sworn positively that the patient was sent from Amherst to him as a man who had a large stone in the bladder, and that he (Dr. Webb) went to Dr. Beaney and told him that it was a large stone, whereupon Dr. Beaney said "The committee will not allow you to operate, as it is against the rules, and therefore I must do the operation myself." One cannot be very sure of a report of a conversation in the operating theatre, where a number of medical students are talking and laughing together, and commenting on the unfortunate wretch about to be operated upon, unless the report is corroborated by substantial facts.

'Far more reliance can be placed on the observations made in reference to this matter by. Dr. Webb, to whom the man was sent for the special purpose of undergoing an operation. In fact, for the very reason given by Dr. Webb, it is impossible that Dr. Beaney can have made the remark, which has been attributed to him, namely that the stone was a small one.

'As to the operation itself, no one will deny that the first part of the operation – the cutting part – was properly done. Nobody attempts to deny it. Even the Coroner will not put that point to you.

The question then arises – when Dr. Beaney discovered that the stone in the bladder was such a large one what should he have done? That is really the turning point in the case, and upon that I will address a few remarks to you.

'Gentlemen, there are two professions in which some accident may arise in the course of a case which must necessitate the immediate use of the judgement of the professional man engaged in that case. These two professions are law and medicine. Gentlemen, it has been my fate – as it is the fate of many members of the bar – to have the life of a man dependent upon my action. Even now I stand before you with a grave responsibility attaching to me, and to every action I take. I may offend the jury by saying one thing; I may please them by another. I must adopt the course, which I think best in my judgement. God forbid I should say I have not made mistakes or that I will not yet make mistakes. Every man makes mistakes. But in surgery, above all things, a man must speedily make up his mind as to what course he will adopt. A successful surgeon has often been described as a lucky surgeon – a man who, at the moment when it is required, has the nerve to do the thing that is right.

'Gentlemen, he may sometimes do the thing that is wrong and he may kill his patient.

'Just put this case to yourselves. Suppose that a medical man is called into a difficult and protracted case of labour. The pains of labour have come on, the child has to be ejected from the womb, and the parts are not sufficient to allow the child to pass. Suppose that Dr. Barker, Dr. Beaney or anybody else, is attending the woman, and that there are two lives dependent upon his action at some point in the labour.

'He tries every endeavour to enable the woman to expel the child, but she is unable to do it; and it comes to the stage that it is absolutely necessary he must do something or the woman will die before his very eyes. He must do something to save either the woman's life or the child's life. It may be that he has to adopt the awful responsibility of destroying one life in order to save the other. Suppose that there is a jealous fellow practitioner looking on, and the accoucheur adopts the responsibility of dismembering the child. Is this jealous practitioner to go next day to the detectives, and say, I would have got the forceps and got the child out; I would have adopted the Caesarean operation, or I would have delivered the woman by some other means? Would any sensible man say that, under such circumstances, the accoucheur should be brought here weeks after the event occurred, that a Coroner's inquest should be held, and that he should be charged with such a serious offence as manslaughter?

'Gentlemen, when Dr. Beaney arrived at the point that he found a difficulty in extracting the stone from the bladder, how do you know in what way the calculus presented itself? Did he know after the first ten minutes or half an hour that it was such a large stone as it proved to be? Is it not likely that it may have presented itself in this way? [exhibiting the stone to the jury with the smallest end foremost]

'If he got hold of it as my fingers now hold it, the first portion of the stone that would be visible would deceptively suggest that it was by no means such a large stone as it really is. It is said that when Dr. Beaney discovered that the stone was a very large one, he ought to have crushed it. In the first place, how was he to crush it? Would this thing (holding up the largest hospital lithotrite) crush it?

'I say, No. Moreover, the operating surgeon had to crush this calculus in a man's contracting bladder. The bladder was empty, there was no urine in it; it was contracting like a glove, pressed down by the lower intestines, and kept up on the other hand by a rectum filled with hard faeces. Now what does Erichsen, the great authority, state as to operating in cases of large stone?

> The second plan, which is crushing the calculus in the bladder through the wound in the perineum, would certainly be a hazardous procedure.'

At this stage Purves picked up one of the textbooks and opened it at a marked page.

'There is a special instrument, which has been invented for that purpose, as you will see by the engraving, which I hold in my hand. It is a forceps with a drill in the centre, so that the drill may go through the stone, and split it and break it up. This forceps is now in use but there is not such a one in the Melbourne Hospital, nor perhaps anywhere in Melbourne. However, even with this instrument, Erichsen says:

> ...Crushing the calculus in the bladder, through the wound in the perineum, would certainly be a hazardous procedure. The irritation that would necessarily be set up by the large lithotrite or crusher that has been invented for this purpose, by the presence of the fragments of stone, and by the necessary difficulty and delay of clearing them out of the bladder, would probably be fatal to the patient.

'Dr. Beaney, in performing the operation finds out that the calculus is of uncommonly large size; and he has to exercise his best judgment in this emergency. He has read Erichsen, and he knows that to crush the stone - even if there had been an instrument at hand for the purpose - would be a hazardous procedure. He therefore says that he would sooner try, by slow dilatation, to pull the stone through.

'How can you get over the authority of Erichsen, that to have tried to crush the stone would have been a hazardous procedure, and probably have proved fatal to the patient? It is impossible to get beyond that point, for Erichsen is one of the greatest authorities on the subject. Dr. Beaney exercises his best judgement. He says, I won't crush it. He knows that it will probably be fatal to the patient to crush it, and he says, I will use my judgment, and Erichsen goes on to state:

> In the event of it being impossible to extract the calculus through the perineum, I think it would

be safer to adopt the third course, and to perform the recto-vesical operation.

'Now the recto-vesical operation, and Lloyd's operation, which Dr. Beaney performed, are twin brothers. It is said by two or three of the witnesses that Dr. Beaney stated, before he commenced the operation, that he would do the median operation, because the stone was a small one. How is that compatible with his action the day before? What did he do on the previous day? Why, he went into the dead house, where there were two dead subjects, on which he rehearsed an operation, with a view to the very operation he was about to perform on the patient Berth. He made the students place their fingers in the wound, which he cut – what for? Why, in order that they might be convinced, by actual touch, that the space obtained by the bi-lateral operation would afford no more room than that obtained by the median operation which he intended to adopt on the living patient. Clearly he was anticipating that he would need as much room as he could possibly obtain to remove the stone.

'Gentlemen, does not the fact that Dr. Beaney went and practised the operation beforehand show some amount of care and some anxiety to perform the operation successfully, and to the best of his ability? Although he may have performed the operation 20 or 30 times before, yet he determined to rehearse it on a dead body before performing it on this occasion.

Why, this is proof palpable that he was endeavouring to do his best in the case.

'Now, gentlemen, with regard to the course, which should have been adopted in connection with this stone, let us see what some of the authorities suggest. Erichsen says there is absolute danger in crushing the stone, although a new and powerful lithotrite has also been invented for the purpose of crushing the stone. Well, nothing of the sort was at hand, and Dr. Beaney was obliged to do the best he could in order to meet the great difficulty, which confronted him. What did he do, and what did Dr. Webb do? They got hold of the two scoops – one was placed under the stone in this fashion, and the other was put over the stone in this fashion (illustrates his remarks by taking the two scoops and placing one above and the other below the calculus). There is only evidence of the bending of one scoop. When Dr. Beaney and Dr. Webb got hold of the stone with these two scoops they levered it out. Great stress has been laid by the Coroner upon the fact that these scoops were merely surgical spoons, and not intended to be bent.

'I do not like to obtrude my knowledge against that of the Coroner, who is a man of great experience in such matters, and he certainly knows a spoon when he sees one; but I beg to differ from him on this question, and I will show you that there is a very important distinction between them and mere spoons. If you try them you will find that both of these instruments have a number of saw-like teeth.

'What in the name of common sense are those teeth for, if not for holding purposes? Put your fingers into them and you will find that they hold [extending the instruments for several of the jurors to see and to feel their edges]. They are also for pulling purposes, and one of the witnesses said that he would use them for such. It is distinctly and positively in evidence that before these scoops were used, Dr. Beaney had succeeded in getting the stone so that his finger could touch it. If that were the case, the stone must have been near the orifice of the wound. What more harm, then, could there be in using the scoops than in using an instrument which may be described as a pair of spoon forceps? Much importance has been attached to the fact that one of the scoops was bent, and it is said that great force must have been used to bend it. I am not a strong man – I don't suppose there is a man in this room who is not stronger than I am – and yet I bent this scoop yesterday as if it were a bit of an old teaspoon. There it is, gentlemen; you can try it yourselves (handing one of the scoops to the jury foreman). Again, according to Mr. Jones, the instrument-maker, it only required a weight of 25lb to bend it.

'Was there any uncommon force used with the scoops? Even if there was, do we not find that uncommon force is sometimes absolutely necessary? From Erichsen it appears that in every operation for stone, if the stone be of the size of a marble up to two inches in circumference, it is absolutely necessary to use force. And, gentlemen, I think I can explain how that is the case.

'When you have cut down to the prostate gland, in the way illustrated by the picture I showed you yesterday, and when you have passed through that, you get to a circular ring, like an india-rubber ring, which tightly closes the neck of the bladder. This ring, or sphincter, contracts, so as to close the orifice after the urine is voided.

'The prostate gland, which is a sort of key to the bladder, is not much bigger than a walnut. Through that gland has got to come the stone, just as does the urine flow through the voiding tube, which passes down the centre of the prostate gland. Instruments and operations have been invented simply to enable the passage of large substances through the neck of the bladder, through the prostate gland and out of the wound made for the purpose of extracting it. It stands to reason that it is impossible to get any stone out of the bladder – I don't care what size the stone is – without dilatation of the prostate gland. Now dilatation means laceration and tearing, according to Erichsen. I take him as an authority. Dilatation is a comparatively modern invention. Formerly it was necessary to cut, and cutting has been again adopted; but it is a "vexata questio" amongst surgeons as to which method they should adopt-whether they should cut or dilate. Upon this vexed question each surgeon has a right to make his own decision. Beaney may prefer dilatation; Moloney may prefer cutting. It is a mere question of experience and of judgement. I will read to you what dilatation means. Erichsen states it in much fewer words and in much better language than I can:

> So in the median operation, the prostate may be dilated to a considerable extent without opening into its capsule. I have used the word 'dilate', but dilatation appears to me to be an erroneous term. I believe that the prostate is not simply dilated, but partially lacerated.

'Now, a great surgeon, in writing on this subject, says it would be both cruel and dangerous to adopt the process of dilatation. That, however, was in the old days, before the discovery of chloroform, when stretching of the parts must have been accompanied by the most terrible and excruciating pain. I can imagine that the agony of a man undergoing that operation, and the parts being dilated by the opening forceps or by the fingers, must have been so horrible that it was necessary to give up that portion of the operation and adopt cutting. But nowadays, when the operation, owing to the grand discovery of chloroform is a painless one, dilatation is again in vogue amongst a great number of surgeons. I am not to determine, nor are you, which is the better system. Doctors differ, and when doctors differ, it is not for a jury to say which is right. Both are done-there is no doubt about that. Let me remind you again what Erichsen says:

> I have often examined the prostate in the dead subject, after it has been subjected to this process of 'dilatation' and have always found its substance more or less torn. A laceration of the substance of the prostate, however, is of no consequence, and only becomes dangerous when it amounts to rupture of the capsule, when it exposes the patient to the fatal accident of extravasation of urine and diffuse inflammation of the pelvic fascia.

'He goes on to say under the heading of Manipulation of the Forceps and Extraction of the Stone:

> In the adult, the main difficulty of lithotomy does not lie in entering the bladder, but in the completion of the operation, that for which the operation has been undertaken – the removal of the stone. And the difficulty and danger increase in proportion to the size of the calculus.

'Supposing that Dr. Beaney, by diagnosis, had discovered that the calculus was only two inches in diameter, that he adopted the median operation, and that, having opened the bladder he found there was a projection in the calculus which made it two and a quarter inches in diameter. Would it be dangerous to dilate?

'Do you mean to say that he would not be justified in dilating to the extent of a quarter of an inch, when every textbook and writer on the subject lays it down that you can dilate these parts without danger, and that such lesions are not the most dangerous accidents?

'By a lesion I mean a wound, which is not the result of cutting but of dilatation or tearing, and one of the authorities says that such lesions are by no means dangerous. Erichsen goes on to say:

> The tissues between the neck of the bladder and the perineal integuments must either be widely cut, or extensively torn and bruised, to allow the passage of a large stone ... A calculus, for instance, two inches in diameter, cannot be extracted by the median operation without the employment of great violence.

'Well, gentlemen, there is no doubt that great force was used in this instance. But the question is – for after all it comes to this – do you suppose that Dr. Beaney, a man whose whole reputation depends upon his skill in these cases, would absolutely go to the trouble of sending out invitations to people to come and witness his operation if he did not intend to perform it to the best of his ability. With enemies and friends there – particular enemies – all watching him at his work, do you suppose that he would be such a bungling idiot, to use the plainest language, as to jeopardise his position by doing anything that he did not think was for the best in such an operation? He was there as a teacher, and he did his very best. There is no doubt about it. No one can doubt that he might have pulled the stone out by force; but the time that elapsed is a sufficient indication of his care and anxiety in the matter.

'What says Dr. Webb? He says that Dr. Beaney was working and working – that he tried every method in his power to get the stone out. That shows some care. How long did the operation last? Taking the compunction of the young gentlemen who have been examined as against that of an experienced practitioner like Dr. Dempster – supposing their estimate of the time to be correct – the longer the time Dr. Beaney was, the more care he used in trying to extract the stone. There can be no doubt about that.

'It is said, and it is alleged to be a vital point in this case against Dr. Beaney, that he did not have a consultation before he performed this operation. Now just let us look at this matter – let us grasp this difficulty, if it be a difficulty, which I deny. What are really the facts? This man Berth has been in the Amherst Hospital for 18 months out of the three years that he had been known to be suffering from stone. A letter came to Dr. Webb, who went to Dr. Beaney, and said, 'I have a man coming from the Amherst Hospital to be operated upon for stone if he can get a bed in the Melbourne Hospital.' The diagnosis was made at Amherst. It was proved beyond the possibility of a doubt, so far as tests could prove it, that the patient was suffering from stone, and he came to Melbourne, and afterwards went to the Melbourne Hospital. Dr. Annand there passed a sound and caused him excruciating agony – such agony that he was forced to shout out.

'Dr. Beaney went afterwards, and, knowing nothing about the prior sounding, he examined the patient and found there was a stone. In view of the operation he was about to perform, he went straight off to the dead house; and there, in the presence of a number of students, experimented to see how he could get the most room in order to reach the stone.

'Is it common sense to suppose that, at that moment, Dr. Beaney did not know that the patient had a comparatively large stone? But what man, in the practice of his profession, could ever suppose that such a monstrous deposit as this was to be discovered? What more did Dr. Beaney do? There are four honorary surgeons, and he caused notices to be sent to the other three that the operation was to be performed. How many appeared there to assist him in the operation? Not a single one.

'What does that indicate? You know quite sufficient of the unfortunate events that disturb the calm atmosphere, or what should be a calm atmosphere, of the Melbourne Hospital – how petty jealousies and squabbles are engendered there; and what do they eventuate in? Inquests. That is what they come to. One squabble has burst – has culminated in this inquest. What does it proceed from? Ill-feeling and, it may be, from jealousy. Your attention has been called to a rule of the hospital. Now let us see what that rule really says. It states that: 'No important operation in surgery...' Dr. Barker says lithotomy is not an important operation – that he can do it in three minutes on an average 'shall be performed without the previous consent of the patient, if in a position to give it...' Well, this man was sent to the Hospital for the very purpose of being operated upon for stone, 'nor unless sanctioned, on a consultation, by two at least of the surgeons...' How on earth was that sanction to be obtained in this case? 'except in cases of emergency'. Why the man was sent to Melbourne to be operated upon for stone! He was crawling about the hospital grounds, bent double with the awful pain he was suffering, passing bloody matter through the penis, and unable to void urine except in small gushes. It was stopped by this enormous mass of stone in his bladder. Was this not a case of emergency? The poor wretch was suffering from retention of the urine, and his kidneys and other delicate parts were affected. Surely it was a case of emergency to relieve a man from such a state of suffering as this.

'But suppose that Dr. Beaney did not hold a consultation. Suppose that he broke this rule. I believe that nearly all the rules of the hospital are only observed in the breaking of them, as a general thing. If you look at the proceedings of the Hospital Committee, you will see that every week new rules are being proposed, observations are made on the breaking of the rules, cases are brought before the committee, concerning young gentlemen at the hospital not keeping the prescribed hours and so forth, and innumerable censures are passed. Admitting, however, for the sake of argument, that Dr. Beaney did break the rule as to consultations, is that a reason why you should find him guilty of manslaughter? The thing is preposterous. It may be a proper subject for investigation by the Committee, or for censure by them, but it is ridiculous that it should be made a reason for the holding of this inquest. Do you mean to say that if there had been a consultation the result would have been different? Do you suppose that, even if the man had been operated upon by Dr. Barker, the man who can beat Erichsen, Cooper, and all the other great surgeons – Dr. Barker, who never fails to detect a stone – it would have made an iota of difference in favour of the man? Did this man's life depend upon a consultation? If it did, he had that consultation at Amherst. The man was sent down to Melbourne specifically to be operated upon for stone, from which disease he had been suffering for years. Can it be said that there was any necessity for a consultation, any such necessity as there would be in a case in which doubt existed as to whether an operation ought to be performed or not? It may have been a breach of the hospital rules not to have had a consultation, but I do not attach any significance to that. That portion of the case is a mere drop in the bucket.

'The real question is, what amount of force, or, to use the very unpleasant word that the Coroner put into every doctor's mouth, what amount of levering was used to get the stone out of the bladder? The Coroner is no doubt fond of mechanical studies, and insists that the stone was got out by leverage. In reality, however, it was not leverage, but simply pressure. You can see for yourselves, gentlemen, that it was pressure that was used. Holding the stone between the two scoops you may use a force of 100lb weight, and no damage will be done except that the scoops will be bent. The stone was held up by one strong man and pressed down by the other, in order to get a firm grasp of it. By pulling it up gently, after having grasped it firmly, the stone slipped out. Do you mean to tell me that Dr. Webb and Dr. Beaney could not have pulled the stone through the perineum without difficulty, if they had chosen to use sufficient force? But they did not try to do so. They simply tried to guide the stone.

'It is complained that the stone was levered out instead of being crushed; but could it have been crushed by any of the instruments in the hospital? The young gentleman in charge of the instruments says that he crushed a piece of bluestone metal with one of the lithotrites, but I would like to know what sort of metal it was, where it was picked from, what shape it was, and whether it would not crush and split like a bit of loaf sugar. But, gentlemen, do you suppose that it was possible to break up this stone in the bladder? The very turning of the screws of the instrument, opening up and may be tearing the bladder and the peritoneum, would make the procedure hazardous.

'What do the textbooks say as to crushing a large stone in the bladder? What does Erichsen say? Why, he says that in most cases it would be fatal! [emphasises this last word]

'When the critical time came, when it was absolutely necessary that Dr. Beaney should make up his mind as to what should be done in the emergency, one of the bystanders brought him this lithotrite [Purves again picked up a lithotrite] this thing, which I call a toy. It is not adapted for such a purpose. There is, however, an instrument for crushing large stones in the bladder. It is a strong forceps – a very powerful instrument, with a drill that will go right through the stone and so break it up. Suppose that you were in the operating room, surrounded with students all eagerly gazing at you. There is the table, the blood is accumulating below, and the patient is lying on the table almost on the verge of death. Every man who lies on the operating table is almost within the valley of the shadow of death. It may be your province to pull him back again from that valley; or, by some unfortunate mistake or accident, you may send him into eternity.

'That is the most serious responsibility, and in the midst of it you are brought this toy with which to crush the stone. What man would trust his life to it? Would anyone? Would any surgeon try to crush a calculus like this with such an instrument? Supposing the stone would split, which it would not, what would have been the result if it had been split? Why, there would have been jagged pieces of stone and bits of splinters scattered all through the bladder.

'It is true that portions of the soft outside covering of the stone came off with the forceps. Doubtless, Dr. Beaney supposed that he was reducing the stone by means of the forceps, but it turned out that the stone was altogether too large to be crushed. Gentlemen, was there any culpable and criminal negligence on the part of Dr. Beaney, in the desperate difficulty which he had to encounter, in not using the thing which was brought to him? Why, every doctor who suggested the crushing of the stone admitted that it was not a proper instrument for the purpose.

'Dr. Barker says he has got a proper instrument at home, but he did not produce it here when he gave evidence. He also said that there are six lithotrites at the hospital, and that three or four of them are capable of crushing this stone. Now the one that was handed to Dr. Beaney was the strongest of the lot and not one unprejudiced surgeon who has been called says that it was suitable for the purpose. If he did not crush it, what was he do? That is the question, which has been asked of different surgeons, and each one has returned a different answer.

'One aspiring surgeon said he would have adopted the suprapubic operation. Now you must remember that there was an immense wound – a wound necessary for the purpose of the median operation – in the man already; and he had been cut through and dilated; and having suffered all this dreadful operation, which must produce subsequent and consequent disorder in those parts, what is it that some think should have been done when the difficulty of extracting the stone arose? Why, that the man was to be further cut across the lower part of the belly, at the risk of injury to a most delicate substance – the only portion of man's body, which cannot be wounded without great danger and almost certain death. That, again, does not commend itself to your common sense.

'There was an objection to the suprapubic operation, which could not be rectified. All the text writers and all the authorities on the subject say that this operation must be performed with a full bladder. Now this man's bladder was empty and could not be filled. One young doctor said "But in this case you would be able to push the peritoneum to one side." In order to do that you would have to cut right down through the outside flesh until you got to the delicate membraneous tissue, which covers the bowels and the whole of the cavity that the intestines occupy.

'A wound in that membrane is said by the authorities to be one of the most dangerous wounds, which can be inflicted upon the human body. After the whole of the operation seemed likely to prove successful, at any rate in Dr. Beaney's humble judgment, was he then, on the very threshold of success, to turn back and adopt an operation he did not believe in – one that he did not believe to be suitable for the purpose for which it was to be applied? If a surgeon every time he performs an operation, is to be surrounded by jealous men, with notebooks in hand, watching everything he does and if by any misadventure or mistake the patient dies, the police are to be communicated with and he is to be charged with manslaughter, it will be absolutely impossible for any surgeon to conduct an operation.

'What would a surgeon's feelings be under such circumstances? Would he dare to have anything to do with a difficult operation? If, at a time when the operating surgeon requires all his coolness and collectedness the fact were to be present in his mind – and could imperil the success of the operation – that if he made a mistake he would be liable to prosecution for manslaughter, which would be one of the most fearful things which could happen to a person. A man must make mistakes. God forbid that a surgeon should, on account of any mistake or accident, be liable to be charged with manslaughter.

'Now, gentlemen, what did the man Berth die of? Not one doctor has told you, and yet you, by your verdict, have to say what the cause of death was. Now, the causes of death in connection with the operation of lithotomy are manifold. Dr. Neild, although he actually came here to prove to you the cause of death, when I asked him how many causes there were of death ensuing after lithotomy, refused to answer the question.

'He did not come here to be asked such questions as that. He knew all about the matter, but he refused to tell me. I wanted an answer to the question for your information and for mine. The causes of death consequent upon the operation of lithotomy are manifold. It is almost impossible to estimate them. It is said in one book that lithotomy is hedged round with innumerable causes of death.

'In Holmes's *Surgery* there are tables showing the different causes of death in a number of cases, in which lithotomy has ended fatally [picks up the relevant text]. This work says:

> Respecting the difficulties encountered in the extraction of stone, they are almost innumerable, and must be met according to circumstances...

'Some surgeons, more especially recently, have recommended the crushing and breaking up of a large calculus by a lithotrite, or strong crushing forceps, or cutting it in two by appropriate instruments, and then extracting. This has been performed successfully, but great danger and risk is necessarily incurred, for the bladder is generally firmly contracted on the stone, so that the coats and mucous membrane can hardly escape injury. From a table giving the causes of death in ninety fatal cases, you will see how manifold the causes of death are: *Infiltration of urine into cellular tissue of the pelvis, resulting in inflammation* was the cause of death in twenty-two of the cases.

'In this case there was no inflammation of the cellular tissue of the pelvis. According to Dr. Neild's statement, there was actually some fluid in the cavity of the pelvis, a portion of which was taken away. Dr. Williams removed it, but although he and Dr. Neild and Dr. Barker put their heads together, in order to show how very serious this case might be made to appear, the liquid was never brought here, nor was a word said about it. Would there not have been an absolute analysis of it if that would have told against Dr. Beaney? Of course there would. As you now know that fluid had simply accumulated during the postmortem. Amongst the other causes of death given in this table are three from accidents. It is impossible to conceive that there should not be accidents in surgery. Supposing that, after a staff has been put in the wound, and the knife in the groove of the staff, some slight thing pushes the knife out of the groove, and you cut the wrong part – is a surgeon to be charged with carelessness, negligence, manslaughter, or murder, in consequence of an accident of that sort? Why, if that were the case, surgery would have become impossible. Professor Humphry, the leading man of Cambridge in my day, and a great surgeon, once actually ruptured the bladder to such an extent that the stone went right through into the man's body.

Yet that awful rupture was an accident, and no one ever heard of such a thing as an inquest being held on the man's body, or any recommendation that proceedings should be taken against Dr. Humphry.

'Dr. Humphry, perhaps, was not a man who had succeeded in getting on the surgical staff of a hospital, and thereby exciting the opposition of the Barkers and Neilds of the profession.

[Still reading from Holmes's surgical text he continues]

> Amongst the causes of death in the other cases three remained uncertain.

'Gentlemen, you are asked to determine a thing, which the great men by whom these cases have been recorded – such men as Dupuytren, Bryant, Teale, Humphrey and Barnard – actually could not determine the cause of death.

'In one case the patient collapsed – fainted away into the next world. In the work from which I have quoted this table, it is stated that

> Dr. Humphry records one case of great interest, in which, although but little force was used, the bladder was ruptured by the forceps, and the stone escaped through the laceration into the peritoneal cavity.

'The stone, in fact, went out of the man's bladder into his belly. This is called a case "of great interest", and no doubt it is probably regarded in that light by the profession, for, dreadful as the accident was, such cases afford information, which is for the benefit of our common humanity.

'I will now, gentlemen, call your attention to the evidence of Dr. Neild. What is that evidence, and how was it given? Dr. Neild is a gentleman who objects to being cross-examined. He objected to me cross-examining him. He comes here with his evidence all cut and dried. He and Dr. Barker have put their heads together, and the result is brought here in black and white. Dr. Neild is put forward to read it to you, and Dr. Barker is asked, "Do you concur in it?" I once knew a learned judge who obtained for himself a great reputation for ability because he invariably concurred with his brother judges, but he never gave the reason why.

'Dr. Barker concurred with Dr. Neild, who refused to be cross-examined; and what chance had I of eliciting further information from these gentlemen? The very evidence that Dr. Neild refused to be cross-examined about, Dr. Barker concurred in. How could I cross-examine Dr. Barker about what Dr. Neild could not be cross-examined upon? It was a case of 'Codlins and Short'[9] – one was the physician and the other the surgeon. I could not cross-examine Dr. Neild, because he would not answer me.

---

9 from The Old Curiosity Shop by Charles Dickens

'He wondered at me, a mere barrister, assuming to come here to talk to him, a physician, who knew all about surgery, but would not tell us anything. I asked him why he showed so much temper, and he replied that he had no interest in the case. No one ever supposed that he had. He only represents one clique, and Dr. Beaney may represent a clique of his own. Dr. Neild examined the body. He had the gratification of seeing this dreadful mass of putrefaction, which had been buried three weeks, and which would never, in the ordinary course of circumstances, have been exhumed.

'If Dr. Barker had performed this operation, I don't think that you would have been troubled to come here.

'If any other man than Dr. Beaney had performed the operation, would there have been an inquest? I am justified in assuming that there would not. I put it to you that there is something in this view of the case. If it had not been for the letter written by A Practical Surgeon there never would have been any such investigation. It has been endeavoured to be shown that Dr. Webb was the cause of this inquest, but that attempt is a lamentable failure.

'Owing to the penuriousness of the Government, who start an inquiry of this kind, and then will not send counsel here to look after it – which seems to me a most monstrous proceeding – the Coroner intimates that he has to perform the functions of a Crown

Prosecutor, as well as those of Coroner. At his instance, a detective is called to contradict Dr. Webb, upon whose statements the whole of these proceedings are said to have been taken.

[At this juncture the Coroner warns Purves to tread warily on this issue, but Purves continues]

'Detective Duncan said that he had an interview with Dr. Webb, that he put a number of questions to him and that to those questions Dr. Webb replied yes. But that is a very different thing from making a statement, which is written down and signed, as the evidence that Dr. Webb has given at this inquest has been. What did Detective Duncan know about peritonitis, lithotrites, lithotomy, or dilatation for stone? Why, all that had been pumped into him before he saw Dr. Webb. The detective went to Dr. Webb, and asked him if he would answer a few questions. He had got the questions ready to put to him pit-pat.

'Dr. Webb, in the innocence of his heart, answered the questions, and said that he was only a lieutenant in the matter. Perhaps he did not know that Duncan was a detective; and, when he did find that out, he wanted to get rid of him, as he did not like to have spies about his house. If Dr. Webb's evidence is to be believed, the Coroner at once should admit that there is no case at all against Dr. Beaney; but he endeavours to break down Dr. Webb's evidence. He implies that it is untrue, and he gets Detective Duncan to say what Dr. Webb's evidence should be.

[Again the coroner intervenes with 'I warn you, Mr. Purves.']

It was clear however that Dr. Youl felt hamstrung by his role both as Prosecutor and Coroner and felt that as the former he probably must allow Purves to address his (Dr. Youl's) handling of the enquiry.

'Is it fair to bring a man here on a charge of manslaughter, and afterwards to turn round and charge one of the witnesses in the case with perjury? That, however, is on a piece and parcel with the whole of this investigation. Dr. Neild, in his written statement, says:

> There was a wound with roughened edges in the perineum in the middle line of the body. It extended forward from the back of the fundament. Its length was 37/8 inches and at its greatest breadth 1 3/4 inches. A probe introduced at the upper part of this wound, and pressed downwards, passed freely into the rectum.

'From the drawing which you saw yesterday you know it is absolutely necessary that there should be a passage into the rectum, in order to get room to extract the stone. It is called the recto-urethral operation. It means that the rectum is to be cut. In the course of getting the stone out – in the course of dilatation, which means laceration – this cut is forced wider open; or, in other words, it tears. In protracted labours, where there is a difficulty in getting the child from the parts, this frequently happens.

'If you ask the first accoucheur you meet whether in his experience he has ever known extensive laceration of the rectum, he will tell you that he not only knows one case but many cases, and that the patients have recovered. The books say that such a lesion is not necessarily fatal; there must be something else to cause death. Now, when Dr. Neild made the post-mortem examination, what state was the body in? It was putrefied and swollen, swollen with gas and in a state of active decomposition. He says in his previous report, which cannot be cross-examined, because he will not let me cross-examine him upon it, that there were ragged edges to this wound. Directly putrefaction set in, these soft parts would become softer and softer. They would become quite friable, and the edges would necessarily crumble away. This does not take place all at once, but gradually, like a bit of ice melting in the summer's sun. Do you mean to tell me that the wound would have presented the same appearance three weeks after the body had been buried that it did when it was first made?

'If there was to be an inquest, why was not the inquest held at the time that the man died? If Dr. Williams, who was at the operation, made notes and communicated with the detectives, why, in the name of goodness and common sense, did he not take the lithotrite and crush it if he believed that ought to be done in order to save the man's life? Why did he not say – I will not stand by and see the man murdered? He did not do anything of the kind but he went away to his private room, wrote out his notes, and caused them to be filtered through Dr. Webb, by the help of Detective Duncan, and Dr. Beaney is brought here to gratify some spirit of I do not know what.

'Perhaps it is in order that Dr. Williams may force his own way up the ladder while another man is forced down. How do we know what his objective was? We do know that Dr. Barker and Dr. Neild went away from the post-mortem without giving notice to Dr. Beaney that they were going to hold a secret meeting with Dr. Williams at Dr. Barker's house. At that meeting some of the parts of the body were further examined, and the whole of the evidence of the post-mortem was arranged. That is not the way in which inquiries should be conducted in order to arrive at the truth between man and man. It savours rather of getting up a criminal prosecution.

'The Coroner, who himself is a physician, gets hold of lecturers at the University, who come here with prepared statements which cannot be properly cross-examined. These men – Dr. Barker, Dr. Neild, and Dr. Williams – apparently meet together in order that they may try and shake Dr. Beaney from the eminence that he has climbed to; or, to adopt the expressive phrase used upon one occasion by Mr. Francis, late Chief Secretary of the colony, to "throw him over the top of the monument", in order that some mere pigmy practitioners may climb up into his place.

'Now was the patient, Berth, a healthy subject? Had he any organic disease? Dr. Neild's own report shows that he was a subject upon whom, of all men, the operation of lithotomy was likely to be dangerous and almost inevitably fatal. It says: "There were some old adhesions of the peritoneum at the lower portion of the large intestine."

'This at once shows that there was some lurking disease, which no surgeon, however able, could determine. It was a disease of this kind, which killed one of the greatest men of modern times. It is a disease that it is absolutely impossible, by any diagnosis known to the medical profession, to determine whether it exists or not. This disease in all probability did exist in this unfortunate man. It is known by the technical name of 'surgical kidney'.

'"Surgical kidney" is like a slumbering and smoldering fire lying at the seat of a man's life, which may be stirred up by the slightest operation.

'By the simplest thing the fire may be kindled which will burn out the man's life. Perhaps the act of Dr. Annand, in passing a sound into the bladder, was the very first thing that stirred up this fatal disease, surgical kidney in this unfortunate man.

'What is Dr. Neild's statement in regard to the kidneys? He says "The left kidney, on one section, was seen to be of a deep claret colour." Think of a kidney in that state. The left ureter, especially at its entrance into the bladder, was much congested.

'The ureter is an organ in the immediate vicinity of the kidney – the tube from the kidney to the bladder – which frequently is a source of disease, and by which stones that form in the kidney sometimes pass into the bladder, causing great disturbance and sometimes resulting fatally. Dr. Neild says "The right kidney was highly congested"; which means, gentlemen, that it was a burning flame at the root of this man's life. Who can tell when that began? Who knows that it may not have been smoldering during the three long years he was suffering from stone in the bladder, and walking about crouched over from the fearful pain that he was suffering. Do you suppose, gentlemen, that this man, walking about with this awful calculus pressing on one of the most delicate and susceptible organs of the human frame, was not prone to death? Is it possible that such a monstrous calculus as this could accumulate in any one corner of the human frame without affecting the whole of it? Some of the witnesses say that the unfortunate man was in good condition, and others say that he was emaciated. Is it possible that he was in a good state of health when it was necessary to remove this huge stone from him? What does Dr. Neild say was the cause of death? "I believe the cause of death to have been shock." And, gentlemen, surgical shock, to use my own language, in these operations, is a very frequent cause of grave apprehension to the operator, and sometimes of death to the patient. Shock has to be met by reviving the energies of the patients with hot bricks, the administration of stimulants, and such other means as were adopted by Dr. Beaney in this case.

'Dr. Neild says

> I believe the cause of death to have been shock from injuries received during the operation, with consequent inflammation of the bladder, ureters and kidneys, and peritonitis.

'We can dismiss peritonitis as a cause of death for we have heard that with peritonitis there is fluid in the cavity and Dr. Neild from his notes agreed that on opening the abdominal cavity there was no fluid. Now, gentlemen, is there the slightest evidence to show that the inflammation of the ureters and kidneys came from this particular wound? May it not have proceeded from the passing of the "sound" by Dr. Annand, or from the sound introduced by Dr. Beaney? Was the cause of death, shock? Was it an accident? Did it result from surgical disease of the kidneys? Did it result from pyaemia? What was it from? Which one of these causes is death attributable to? I think you will say that the operation – in addition to the stone being a large one – was an operation performed on a man who was suffering from a chronic disease at the time it was undertaken.

'Dr. Barker certainly gave his evidence in a more satisfactory fashion than Dr. Neild.

'I must compliment him by saying that, although he showed some temper under cross-examination, it was not of the offensively reticent character of Dr. Neild's. Dr. Barker says he thinks a bigger stone can be taken out by the median than by the lateral operation. Yet he says that he should have adopted the lateral operation. Why, gentlemen, it is a mere question of opinion. I believe that if you were to collect all the surgeons in Collins Street, with a dragnet, and pull them into this building, and ask them their opinion upon the evidence before you, not two of them would agree. They have all got their little idiosyncrasies, just as every man who ever addressed a jury has got his little tricks of rhetoric. They have all got their little knacks. Whether it is a Barker, a Gillbee, or a Beaney, each one has got some little method of performing an operation, upon which he agrees to differ with his fellow practitioners.

'Gentlemen, you have listened to me with great attention, and, in conclusion, I will only address a few further remarks to you. The gravest responsibility in connection with this case, gentlemen, rests upon your shoulders, because you, like a surgeon in the operating theatre of a hospital, have at your command the whole future of a living man. It is not the mere question of destroying the body of a man and allowing his soul to another world. Dr. Beaney may be said to have done that by mistake or by accident, but you gentlemen, by your verdict, may consign a man to a living death.

'There is no doubt about it. If by your verdict you say that Dr. Beaney was criminally negligent; that, in the face of men, and in the open light of day, he so prostituted and degraded the noble profession he is a master of, and forsook the energy and skill he had a right to give to this unfortunate man; if you say that by criminal carelessness and negligence he did away with this man's life, directly you return such a verdict Dr. Beaney is morally damned for ever, his profession is gone from him, he is a pariah and an outcast from his fellow professional men. You have this grave responsibility upon you, and I, gentlemen, have an equally grave one upon me, because I have to stand between Dr. Beaney and those who are pursuing him with such tenacity. Therefore, you must fully understand that I feel the grave responsibility, which devolves upon me to the utmost extent that is possible.

'Gentlemen, I ask you to aid me. You will have the main circumstances of this case placed before you by the Coroner, who, as a medical man, is far more qualified to deal with it than I am, and he will be able to point out to you any little things which may have escaped me, and which may, therefore, seem to your minds to have some force. I ask you, gentlemen, to help me, because you have heard all the evidence, and it is impossible for any one man, be he whom he may – it is impossible for any advocate who may be brought here – to carry in his mind all the numerous points that there are in this most remarkable case. I can only grasp the salient ones.

'When you retire to consider your verdict, if there is any point, which may have escaped me, I hope that you will fully consider it, and not, because an advocate forgets it, think that he has passed it by designedly.

'I am afraid of occupying your time; I know the season of the year, and I am unwilling at any greater length to detain you from your homes. You were brought here I do not know how, or upon what system. You have been apparently brought from all districts – one from each street. The usual rule in summoning a Coroner's inquest is for the Coroner's officer to get together the first dozen or fifteen men he can come across; but I am glad that that plan has not been adopted in this instance, because I see before me a body of men of more than the usual intelligence. I ask you to give me and to give my client the benefit of your assistance.

'It would be preposterous to doubt – there is no doubt – at whom these proceedings are pointed and I stand here as his representative. You can see my brief, gentlemen; it consists of blank paper. I knew nothing of what evidence was to be brought forward. It may be that, had I known what evidence was to be given, I would have brought witnesses here. But what is the necessity for it? When the Coroner is obliged to discredit his own principal witness, and to bring a detective here to say that the evidence that witness gave is not true, what necessity is there for me to call witnesses? You have got the whole facts before you.

'Although it is impossible for me in the few hours, which I have been able to devote to this case to thoroughly master, and bring together all the knowledge, which might be collected from the evidence which has been given, it is perfectly clear from that evidence that Dr. Beaney did not violate one leading principle of surgery. There can be no doubt about that. A mere error of judgment, if there was one, is not to be brought in judgement against him. You are not to say that he committed manslaughter if he made a mistake.

'I think that, on the whole facts of the case, even the authorities of the Crown will admit – I am sure that if they had any mouthpiece here they would admit it – that they have made a mistake in these proceedings.

[The Coroner interrupted Purves again and sharply advised the jury to ignore that last comment. Purves seemed undisturbed and continued.]

'The deceased, when once taken to his long home, ought to have been left there and you ought not to have been brought from your earthly homes, in order to make a protracted investigation as to the cause of his death.

'Gentlemen, these are the remarks that I have thought, in the limited time I have had at my command that I should place before you. Had I had a longer time for preparation I might have made a more elaborate speech. Have I a good case to go to you? I think I have; and that absolves me of much of the responsibility, which I would otherwise feel. I say that this case throughout is a fiasco. Dr. Beaney may walk forth from here, with your verdict in his favour that he is a reliable surgeon, and a fit and honest man to be entrusted with the great functions, which his profession gives him.

He may go back again to that great institution, the Melbourne Hospital, without any ban upon him – with your verdict that he ought not to have faced a criminal charge for what, at the very utmost, was an error of judgement. Criminals are not recruited from such men as he is. He is above that suspicion. In the operating theatre he used his best endeavours, under circumstances of emergency, in order to save the life of the unfortunate patient upon whom he was operating; and I have no doubt that you will absolve him from any negligence or carelessness in the case.'

In summing up the case Dr. Youl emphasised a number of points. Firstly, that such an operation should not have been performed without a consultation, and at that consultation a discussion on whether to cut or to crush the stone could have been held. The jury must decide if the neglect of a consultation was gross and criminal neglect. He indicated that it was readily understandable that the other surgeons did not attend the case, as they would have been acknowledging responsibility for the management in a case they knew nothing about. If the operation had been conducted under their advice it is likely that no inquiry would have been held.

Secondly, as Mr. Beaney had elevated himself to the position of Senior Honorary Surgeon, extraordinary skill and knowledge were expected of him. Had he shown carelessness in this case?

Thirdly, the operation, so far as the cutting was concerned was properly done. The difficulty arose when the stone was found to be so large. He (Dr. Youl) believed that the suprapubic approach could have been safely used. The jury should decide if Dr. Beaney should have used this approach.

Fourthly, Mr. Purves had made much of a doubtful entity called "surgical kidney". Dr. Youl felt that surgical kidney was to the surgeon what a cat was to a servant, the cause of a great deal that she could not account for. He felt that little attempt had been made to ascertain whether there was any disease of the kidney or not.

He stated that it was his belief that the conduct of the inquest had been properly and fairly conducted and he concluded with a reminder that the jury must be satisfied that there was a total disregard of a man's life and that there had been nothing short of culpable and criminal negligence before they could find Dr. Beaney guilty.

The Coroner then directed all except the jury to leave the hearing room. He advised the jury that sustenance would be provided to them and they were to take their time over their deliberations.

The foreman, Mr. Edgar Burton, asked if they could have some illustrations showing the various part of the body relevant to the operation. Burton was a teacher and a Latin scholar. He felt that he had some understanding of the medical jargon but that others of the jury might not. It so happened that there were some anatomical sketches of the abdomen and the male pelvis, both front and side views, in the dissecting room and these were brought in and left with the jury.

10. The verdict and public reaction

Purves had been right in that the all-male jury had to some extent been selected and could be described mainly as educated and therefore also to some extent middle class, if such a thing existed in Melbourne at that time. Amongst the fifteen members of the jury were teachers, public servants, merchants, publicans, tradesmen, a banker and a builder. Apart from the initial annoyance of being away from their families during the holiday period, the jury duty was not taking them away from the earning of income. Thus, apart from the initial horror a number of them felt on viewing the exhumed body, most had settled down to enjoy the experience of seeing and listening to the contest played out before them.

When they were left to themselves, Burton first asked if anyone had not understood the operation. It appeared that two of the public servants and one of the tradesmen were unclear as to what the prostate was and where it was situated. Burton pointed it out in the illustrations of the male anatomy but could go little further than that. There was no one on the jury with more than scant knowledge of anatomy and certainly no one with any knowledge of biology or disease.

Burton then asked if they could agree on the cause of the patient's death and almost everyone started speaking at once, creating quite a cacophony of sound. It caused Burton to call for some order and he suggested that just one voice be heard at a time, and with an orderly progression, as they sat around the table they had moved to after the instruments and textbooks previously displayed had been cleared.

George Sweet, the banker, then spoke first stating that there was a difference of opinion on the cause of death, between peritonitis, claimed by some witnesses and inflammation of the kidneys, raised by the defending barrister and also agreed to by other witnesses as a possibility. Thus he felt that the jury members, as they were not doctors, should not make a deliberation as to the cause of death.

This seemed a sensible suggestion to some but raised eyebrows with other jurors. Leonard O'Keefe, a teacher, asked if this was not a critical issue. 'How can we decide which of the doctor's actions were culpable if we don't know what killed the patient? Was it tearing the rectum? Did that result in peritonitis?'

A clothing merchant, Benny Green, entered the discussion. 'But I thought Purves showed that Berth didn't have peritonitis, when it was agreed that with peritonitis there is always fluid in the cavity and in this case there was no fluid.'

'Yes Dr. Barker was sure he died from peritonitis,' said O'Keefe. 'But do you not see that Barker is biased. Beaney is on the Melbourne Hospital staff and he is not,' countered Green.

Burton let the jurists go on for some time in this more ordered way, but discerning that considerable uncertainty remained in the minds of most of the members, as to exactly what Berth had died from, he brought them back to George Sweet's recommendation that they should not make a statement on the cause of death. After some further discussion there was agreement on this point. Having brought them to this agreement Burton wondered whether the Coroner would accept their decision on this issue. However he felt that they were making progress and he then called for further discussion, questions or comments.

John Retallick, a public servant, asked 'What did Dr. Beaney do that was wrong – should he have crushed the stone?'.

Ian McDonald, one of the tradesmen, knowing the value of having the right tools and recognising Beaney's dilemma, commented that 'There wasn't a suitable instrument in the operating room. The lot which the hospital had was not good enough.'

Frederick Fanning, a fellow tradesman, supported him, 'Aye, you would need a sledge hammer to crush that "brick".'

Taking up this theme a third teacher, Myles Statham, wondered if there wasn't some blame to be attached to the hospital for not having the most up to date instruments available, instruments, which could cope with any emergency or unusual circumstance. Sweet, with his knowledge of the constant hospital practice of soliciting funds for the ever-increasing demand on its services (given the rapidly growing population) responded 'That is probably a matter of funding. I doubt if the hospital could cater for the whim of every surgeon to have special instruments to cover every conceivable difficulty.'

The other merchant, a man named Maddocks, cut in. 'Dr. Beaney's lawyer read such a lot of medical details about operations to us that I found it somewhat confusing.' There were nods of agreement as Maddocks continued, 'So I do not think that we can argue about the operation, just as we cannot argue about the death. If the doctors could not agree on whether he should have continued to cut, or to try to crush the stone, then we are in no position to decide on what he should have done.'

By this stage there was a feeling of frustration amongst the jurors as voiced by Statham. 'If we cannot say what the patient died from, and we cannot decide what Dr. Beaney should have done, then what can we decide upon?'

Corder, another of the public servants, and a man used to following protocol, spoke up. 'I know what he should have done. He should have had a consultation with the other surgeons in the hospital, and in not doing so he broke the hospital rules. It could not have been so urgent a case if Dr. Beaney had time to rehearse the operation he would perform.'

The builder, James Jordon, cut in. 'In my work if we had to abide by every rule of Government or local shire, we would never get a building finished on time. You have to make your own mind up and go for it. That is what I have to do every day.'

'We are not talking about a building,' said Connors, also a public servant. 'We're talking about a delicate operation to save a man's life.'

Corder, who worked in the same offices as Connors and was superior to him, chipped in again, 'Delicate! From the description we were given it did not seem like a delicate operation to me.'

'I mean a dangerous operation,' responded Connors, a little aggrieved. 'Did it not fit into the Rule 7 as a capital operation?'

Hughie O'Riordon, one of the hotel licensees, entered the discussion. 'I don't know that the patient had much of a life anyway. The Doc was trying to relieve the poor wretch's misery. I guess he did at that, although not the way he might have wanted it to end up.'

Fanning spoke again. 'I think you are right on that point. Poor Mr. Berth was too far-gone anyway. I don't think any surgeon could have saved him. When your kidneys are shot your system gets poisoned and that's it.'

The debate about whether or not Beaney should have called for a consultation went on for quite some time, with the three public servants and the three teachers holding firm that he should have done so, and others arguing that the patient was sufficiently ill for the case to be considered an emergency. However, eventually the public servants and the teachers succeeded in winning over most of the jury.

Sensing that there were no further issues to explore, Burton suggested to the group that, whilst they took some of the refreshments offered, he would prepare a statement of their verdict. When he read the statement there was general agreement with it. Although two of the public servants and one of the teachers considered that it did not contain a sufficiently severe censure of Beaney, the majority was accepting of it and eventually that majority reached the required number of twelve.

At the end of one and a half hours of consultation the jury conveyed an indication to the coroner, through a clerk, that they had agreed to the terms of their verdict. By mid-afternoon the coroner, the jury and interested parties had re-assembled in the inquiry room and the foreman of the jury passed a written paper to the coroner.

The Coroner read the document and looking to the foreman said, 'You do not find the cause of death?'.

The foreman answered, 'We are not in a position to agree as to the cause of death. The medical witnesses themselves are not agreed as to that.'

The Coroner responded, 'Very well, then I shall read the verdict. "That the deceased, Robert Berth, died in the Melbourne Hospital on the 5th instant. We are of opinion that evidence has not been brought before us, to prove Mr. Beaney guilty of culpable negligence at the operation. Still, we are of opinion that, had a consultation been held by the honorary surgeons, in all probability other means might have been used in extracting the stone; and we enter our protest against the rules of the Hospital being broken." Is this your verdict, Gentlemen?'

The foreman responded, 'Twelve of the jury agreed to that and three object to it on the ground that it is not strong enough.'

'I want only the verdict of twelve,' said the Coroner.

The proceedings were then terminated.

A delighted Beaney wasted little time in inviting his two legal representatives to accompany him to the Club. Surprisingly his conversation did not dwell upon A Practical Surgeon or other Melbourne Hospital staff members, whom he knew to be hostile to him. Rather, he spoke in praise of Purves and his ability to rapidly eschew the niceties of stone surgery. Purves thanked him for his complimentary remarks but suggested that he might have gone harder against Rule 7.

To this Beaney replied that Rule 7 would continue to be broken and that one day it would disappear. Consultations were held only when the surgeon believed it to be necessary and in the interests of the patients. He advised Purves not to be further concerned and to celebrate the verdict with a glass of champagne. Even more champagne was consumed that night at the People's Theatre in Bourke Street, where the Beaneys and their legal guests enjoyed Struck Oil, starring James Cassias Williamson and his wife Maggie Moore, who had come out from England to perform in that play only, but stayed for forty years.

In the days that followed the inquest, there were numerous reports in the many newspapers of the Colony and also in those of New South Wales. Whilst the *Daily Telegraph* and *The Age* admonished Beaney for not having called a consultation and having underestimated the size of the stone, they and the *Herald* supported the jury finding of no evidence of culpability and considered the main issue to be a hospital one of inter-professional rivalry.

This theme was enlarged upon in succeeding days. For example the *Hamilton Spectator* spoke of Beaney being pilloried by his rivals, the Jamieson and Woodspoint *Chronicle,* of Beaney being a mark for the arrows of malice and envy to be shot at. The Sydney *Evening News* wrote of the case against Beaney as being brought through envy, hatred, malice and all un-charitableness, although how these regional and interstate journalists could be so certain in their views is unclear.

An editorial in *The Australian Medical Journal,* however, clearly did not agree with the verdict, and felt that all that was possible to do had not been done. It referred to the alarming extent of injury both to the bladder and the rectum, sufficient to render death inevitable. It also indicated that some gentlemen who spoke out so confidently before the inquest apparently did not have the courage to state on oath, what they had previously asserted in private. It was scathing in its comments on Purves as a very ill tempered and bad mannered young gentleman and a very callous barrister. It ended with a statement that Mr. Beaney had not come out of the inquest well; he was not to be envied and he could ill afford further such inquiries.

The extraordinary amount of media coverage, and variance in apparent public opinion for and against Beaney, was noted by a number of his friends in the city. They felt that he had been done a gross injustice and that Melbourne owed Beaney an apology. Prominent among these friends was James (later Sir James) Butters, a broker and charity worker of note, the MLC for the North Eastern province and a previous lord mayor. He called upon the current mayor, James Gatehouse to chair a dinner for Dr. Beaney and to help redress the wrong done to him.

Thus about fifty gentlemen of the city sat down to dinner on the evening of Monday, the 24th of January

1876 at the magnificent Clements, a favourite spot with the colony's cricketers. They were a mixture of friends and patients of Dr. Beaney. The Right Worshipful Mayor, James Gatehouse, occupied the chair and towards the end of the meal the usual loyal toast was held. The mayor then called upon James Butters to read an address and propose a toast to their special guest of the evening. Mr. Butters was regarded as a gifted after-dinner speaker and had a strong but pleasant Scottish accent. At this time he was married to the second of his four wives. He read his address as follows:

> To Mr. James George Beaney, F.R.C.S., Honorary Surgeon Melbourne Hospital.
>
> Dear Sir, – The slight testimonial (a silver inkstand), which accompanies this, is the gift of your friends and patients, offered by them for your acceptance, not so much for its intrinsic value as for the means whereby to express their continued appreciation of your high character and great professional skill. These, combined with your numerous charities and the many eminent qualities that you have demonstrated during your long residence in Victoria, have deservedly won you a vast practice, and the esteem and confidence of a large section of the community.
>
> The various annoyances followed by the late attempt to destroy your professional standing and

> reputation (to which you have, by professional envy and jealousy, been subjected), has aroused much sympathy. You may, however, rest assured that the signal failure of that attempt has reversed the intention of its promoters, by elevating you still higher in public opinion, and rendering your position wholly unassailable in the future. With hearty good wishes, and an assurance of the continued respect and confidence of your many friends and patients, we are, etc.

The mayor made the actual presentation of the massive, solid silver inkstand, the front of which was engraved with Mr. Beaney's crest. On its base was the inscription *Presented to James George Beaney Esquire F.R.C.S. Senior Surgeon to the Melbourne Hospital, by a few of his friends in testimony of their admiration of his professional skills as a surgeon and his upright and honourable conduct as a citizen.*

The Mayor remarked, in handing the gift to Beaney, that he fully endorsed every word contained in the address and the inscription. He then called upon the gathering to drink to the long life and continued prosperity of Dr. Beaney.

Dr. Beaney in turn thanked his friends sincerely for the compliment they had paid him and accepted that the hostility of his professional colleagues had most likely not diminished, but ensured, his popularity. Despite their attitudes he undertook to dedicate more and more of his time to administering to the patients of the Melbourne Hospital in the years to come.

Various other toasts, including one to those members of the press, who had been supportive of Beaney and one to the Ladies concluded a very pleasant evening. It was not, however, to be the last controversy, nor last court case, in which this "unassailable" public figure would be involved over the next decade and a half.

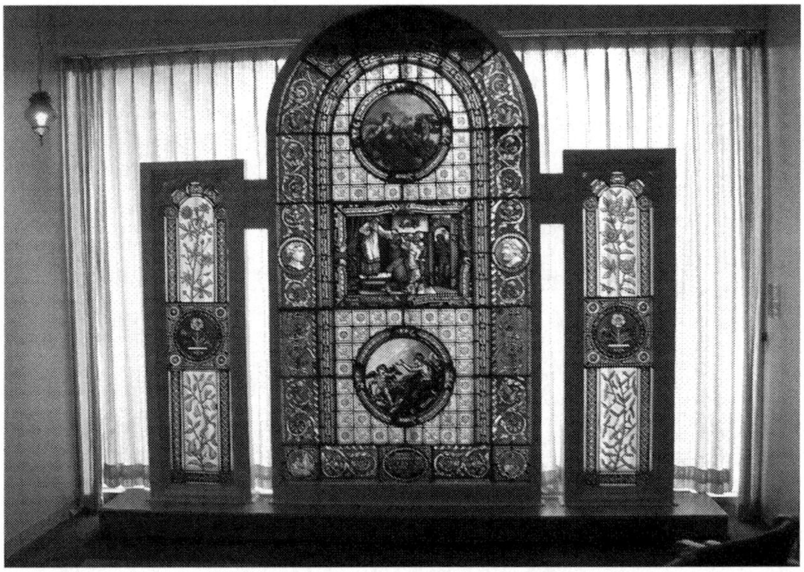

Figure 13: Triptych, donated by James Beaney, Monash Medical Centre, Melbourne.

Epilogue

The reader might wish to know why Robert Berth died. He most likely had poor kidney function and a longstanding urinary tract infection at the time of surgery. The description of the patient on that final evening of putting out little urine, having a rapid pulse with cold limbs and a 'drawn' appearance, suggests that he died from renal failure with septicaemia.

His death was most likely inevitable at that time. Currently, with intensive care, with intravenous fluid support to maintain renal circulation, renal dialysis if required, and antibiotics for the septicaemia, he would have likely survived.

The term "surgical kidney" is not used today but it is still recognised that a patient may become suddenly and severely ill with a septicaemia after instrumentation of the urinary tract. Minor injury to the inner lining of the urethra (voiding tube) may allow entry of bacteria, when subclinical or low-grade infection is already present. This was at risk of occurring when both Doctors Annand and Beaney passed sounds into Robert Berth's bladder on November 30th, just two days before the operation, but there was no way of protecting against it at that time.

In his address to the jury Purves made an important point in quoting Judge Baron Hullock's opinion that

> If a person, bona fide and honestly exercising skill to cure a patient, performs an operation which causes a patient's death, he is not guilty of manslaughter.

Whilst it might seem an obvious statement, without such protection, it is unlikely that developments in surgery in the 19th and 20th centuries would have been so readily accomplished. It does not, of course, prevent a patient or relative bringing an action for negligence against a medical practitioner.

Baron Hullock, incidentally, was the judge who sentenced Edward Gibbon Wakefield, the foundation figure of South Australia, to jail for three years. Wakefield, when he was a young lawyer, had abducted a pretty young heiress called Ellen Turner. He was thirty and she was only fifteen years of age. It was whilst he was in jail for the offence that he studied and developed his blueprint for colonisation, which was later to benefit New Zealand as well as Australia.

Was there an alternative operation, which Beaney should have used at that time? Probably there was not as clearly there was no satisfactory instrument in the hospital with which to crush the stone. Antibiotics were not available to treat peritonitis, which might have occurred if he had used the suprapubic approach, for, as he could not distend the bladder, there was a strong chance that he would have perforated the intestine.

The suprapubic approach would be less hazardous today, even if the bladder could not be distended, for it could be done with antibiotic cover, should the intestine be injured, and the injury to the intestine itself could be repaired, with or without establishing a relieving stoma (bowel bypass).

An alternative modern treatment available now to crush calculi is shock wave lithotripsy and the size of the stone could be determined beforehand by x-ray, as the majority of stones contain calcium and are opaque. However, unfortunately for Robert Berth, as mentioned above, Roentgen's discovery was still twenty years away.

The identity of A Practical Surgeon was never made public. Some clues suggest Barker. The letter demonstrates the writer's knowledge of the then current surgical literature. As Barker was the University Lecturer in Surgery he should, of necessity, have had this knowledge and his professional library was thought to be one of the best in Melbourne. He, of course, was also no friend of Beaney, having been displaced by him at the hospital. A Practical Surgeon had presumed that Berth's death was due to peritonitis and Barker had given evidence that all of his cases that died following this particular operation of lithotomy had done so from peritonitis. In giving his evidence Barker also insisted that the stone should have been crushed, as was the suggestion in the Practical Surgeon's letter. Furthermore the signing of the letter as A Practical Surgeon suggests that the writer possessed a sizeable ego and Barker clearly demonstrated his opinion of his own skills when giving evidence at the inquest.

Although Barker was regarded by Thomas Fitzgerald as the best surgeon in Melbourne in his prime, and at one stage his practice was large, his career was later to be clouded by several unfortunate events and court cases. In 1880 he was replaced by Girdlestone, as the University Lecturer in Surgery, after a student made an accusation (never proven) that he had been drunk while lecturing. He died in 1885 in a state of poverty, having made poor investments and being clouded by multiple court cases. His name lives on, however, for Barkers Road, in the eastern suburb of Kew, is named after the surgeon Edward Barker.

Fitzgerald also remains a possibility as the writer. The patient who underwent the first operation Beaney performed on that fateful December 2nd. was a woman called Ann Kelly. Dr. Annand, the resident, had mentioned in his evidence that she was still alive at the time of the inquest on Berth. She never regained full health however and died on January 29th 1876. She most likely had pulmonary tuberculosis and this was possibly also the problem in her knee. The progress notes at one period recorded that the wound was 'normally suppurating', i.e. that it was infected and pus was being discharged. At the inquest held into her death on February 1st 1876, Mr. Fitzgerald stated that 'It was in his opinion bad surgery to leave this bone as it was left.' The Practical Surgeon had said in his letter, in reference to this particular operation, that 'the cutting had been done poorly and that the amputation had been performed at too low a level, through the problem area of bone.' Hence the Practical Surgeon and Fitzgerald were of the same opinion.

The cause of Mrs. Kelly's death was not clear. Possibly it was due to a combination of pre-existing lung and liver disease plus infection of the amputation stump. The coroner was again Dr. Youl, who found that 'there was no consultation and if there had been the patient in all probability would have survived'. He concluded that there was recklessness but not gross carelessness and the jury determined that she died from the effects of an operation performed by Mr. Beaney. They further determined that he had rushed into operating without a consultation, that he was very rash in performing the operation without consulting the other honorary surgeons and that this practice should be prohibited.

There was much discussion of this case, as well as Berth's, recorded in the minutes of the Medical Society's meeting for February 1876. One might ask if Mr. Beaney was ever going to accept the requirement to involve his peers in decisions about the management of his patients.

Beaney was fortunate in that John Madden, the Minister for Justice in the short-lived McCulloch government of 1875, had allowed him to be represented at the inquest on Robert Berth. Such fairness and courtesy were to attend Madden throughout the rest of his career. He left politics in 1883 and on returning to the bar his success rivalled that of Purves, although his manner was never as aggressive. He was later to become Chief Justice of Victoria, Vice-Chancellor, then Chancellor, of Melbourne University, to receive a knighthood, and finally to be appointed Lieutenant Governor of the State.

In another odd coincidence the surgeon Henry O'Hara, who had purchased Beaney's Cromwell House, and who had assaulted Purves in the street, was raised by Madden's mother, who happened to be his aunt. O'Hara had been orphaned at the age of thirteen and having commenced his schooling at the Jesuit college, Stonyhurst, in Lancashire finished it at Geelong College, where he captained the cricket team.

Was Dr. Beaney a good surgeon? This is difficult to determine in retrospect. He was probably as skilled as most of his colleagues but not in the class of Fitzgerald and James, according to Dr. G.T. Howard, one of Beaney's residents, although he was sometimes daring and successful. The hip operation he attempted to perform on the fifteen-year-old boy Barrie, who died "on the table", is similar to what we know today as a Girdlestone operation or ostectomy,[10] in which a false joint is created, but the Oxford surgeon,

---

10 Ostectomy is removal of bone, osteotomy is cutting of bone.

Gathorne Girdlestone, did not describe it until 1943. Perhaps it was an original idea of Beaney's, as the Practical Surgeon's claim that Dr. Barton of Philadelphia had performed it in 1826 was wrong. Dr. Barton performed an osteotomy* to alter the angle of weight bearing only.

Beaney's rival Barker, from later accounts, was most likely a better surgeon; however, *The Lancet* noted, in his obituary, that Beaney had operated upon 400 patients, to repair hernias, without a death. That would have been quite an achievement in those times, if it were true.

In 1877 there was yet another inquest concerning a patient who died in Beaney's consulting rooms. The male patient presented with a strangulated hernia, which Beaney was trying to reduce, i.e. manipulate the contents of the hernia (usually small intestine) back into the abdominal cavity to relieve the obstruction. The patient died whilst Beaney was still trying to relieve the obstruction. Fortunately for Beaney, evidence was given that the patient had been under treatment for heart disease and a post-mortem confirmed the extent of that disease to be extreme and death therefore not unexpected.

Beaney was clearly very generous with his money, notwithstanding that much of it went to the perpetuation of his own name. His estate was estimated to be around £60,000, an immense fortune in today's terms, and, in addition to the Melbourne

University donations, Beaney presented a beautiful stained glass triptych to the Melbourne Hospital. It is sited today, however, in the nondenominational chapel at the Monash Medical Centre, the connection to that hospital being (as mentioned previously) that the old Melbourne Hospital became the Queen Victoria Hospital, and then the Monash Medical Centre. This explains why the wording on the triptych states 'The gift of James George Beaney, honorary surgeon of this hospital 1878'.

As mentioned in the Introduction he funded The Beaney Institute for the Education of the Working Man in Canterbury, England, the town in which he was born. The original Tudor Revival building still stands today, functioning as a museum and library and known to the locals simply as the "Beaney". As recently as 2012, £14 million was spent by the City of Canterbury in refurbishing it. It is in High Street on the site of an establishment he probably frequented as a young man, the old George and Dragon Inn.

Beaney left money to the Canterbury Cathedral, on one wall of which there is a grouping of five related marble relief plaques, one bearing the inscription "Sacred to the memory of The Hon. James George Beaney MD". He left money also to Guys and St. Thomas's hospitals in London and to all of the Melbourne hospitals then existing. This last bequest was apparently £30,000 to be shared by eight hospitals, in differing amounts.

The illnesses, to which his death is ascribed, namely a cerebral condition complicating liver disease and gout, would appear to confirm his overindulgence in alcohol. He once boasted to a friend that he was continental in his habits, commencing with a bottle of claret at breakfast, a small bottle of "fizz" for lunch and a big bottle for dinner. He was referred to at one time in the Melbourne Medical Record as "Champagne Jimmy". Perhaps he needed it to sustain him through the many more turbulent years, which followed.

His wife died whilst they were abroad in 1879. They had only been married nine years.

Court cases continued to plague him. His publisher Ballière sued him in 1880 over an unpaid debt. The brilliant Purves again defended him successfully, although much came out about Beaney's advertising and questionable publications at that trial. It is interesting that Beaney never made any attempt to publicly refute the many accusations of his plagiarism or the accusations about his contract practice (fee bargaining).

A further case involved an action that Beaney took against Thomas Fitzgerald for slander over the Sebastopol "medal" and for claiming that he, Beaney, had bought his Melbourne Hospital appointment.

After some years of trying to enter politics he was finally elected a Member of Legislative Council in 1883, representing North Yarra.

In 1886 there was much criticism in the press of the Melbourne Hospital, because of its high mortality rate from infection. So high was the death rate from erysipelas (a severe skin infection) that Fitzgerald had refused to operate and Dr. Youl, still the Coroner at that time, had stated publicly that patients had 'no greater chance of living in those wards than if they had their throats cut'.

A Parliamentary Committee of Inquiry was established and Beaney managed to have himself appointed chairman of the Committee of Inquiry.

The Parliamentary report, when released, was seen to be a whitewash. It rejected any need to close (or move) the hospital. All that was necessary was to make some building alterations, to limit the number of patients admitted and to transfer a few patients with chronic infections to the country. A hospital move was not in the interests of Beaney, of course, as well as some of his colleagues, who were used to the convenience of the hospital site in Lonsdale Street, so near to Collins Street, where they had their practices.

The following criticism of the Parliamentary report appeared in the *Illustrated Australian News* on the 18/12/1886.

> The select Committee of the Legislative Council appointed to enquire into the alleged insanitary condition of the Melbourne Hospital have presented their report to the Parliament. The decision and

recommendations arrived at are, as might have been expected, entirely in accord with the opinions previously expressed by the Chairman, Dr. Beaney, in his professional capacity. The Committee in effect states that the hospital is, with a few trifling exceptions easily remedied, almost all that could be desired. Its condition, position and management are eminently satisfactory, and by the removal of the central block and some outbuildings, and the limitation of the number of patients received, there is no necessity for the selection of another site. The internal dissensions of officials, the high rate of mortality, the disease impregnated walls, are mere delusions, while the "scare" which recently existed was the result of exaggerated statements, 'intensified by the coloured and unwarrantable assertions published from time to time'.

The evidence of Dr. Fitzgerald, Dr. Girdlestone, Mr. James, Dr. Robertson, Dr. Youl and other experts consequently goes for nothing while that of Dr. Hudson of Ballarat, and of some medical small fry picked up promiscuously must be accepted as the infallible truth. It is doubtful whether the public will be satisfied with such a lame and impotent conclusion, and one contrary to every day experience and to common sense. It was simply burking the matter to allow a partisan medical practitioner to act as chairman of the Committee and to throw the whole weight of his representative, no less than his professional

> influence, into the controversy. The Committee was in the main guided by his opinion, so that contrary to the deliberate conclusions of the leading members of the faculty in the colony, the hospital is to remain intact. The only sensible suggestion made. is for the erection of a hospital in the country, for special care of phthisis cases.

The Dr. Hudson of Ballarat, mentioned in the article as supporting the Committee's opinion, was probably Dr. Robert Hudson, who, as also being a founder of the Ballarat Bank, is likely to have been more attuned to issues of finance than infection. It would be more than fifty years before the Melbourne Hospital moved to a new site in Parkville, where it stands today as The Royal Melbourne Hospital and is across the road from the Melbourne University Medical School.

Beaney again caused strife when, using a "doctored" letter of introduction from Graham Berry (written during his time as Victorian Premier), he travelled extensively in America, Europe and the U.K. as an unofficial ambassador. He was feted by hospital boards and was the toast of London society. Beaney weathered the subsequent storms from the Medical Society and the press that greeted his return to Melbourne, as he had done so often in the past. It apparently transpired that Bailliere had altered the letter to read as an 'Honorary Commission' from the Premier.

Not long after the Berth inquest Beaney set about the completion and furbishing of his magnificent house of four stories (and a tower) on the southeast corner of Collins and Russell streets. With his name boldly printed above the door he carried on his practice on the ground floor and entertained often and extravagantly on the first floor and on the roof garden, until his death on 30 June 1891. Apparently two weeks beforehand he accurately predicted the day and the hour of his death. As mentioned earlier, the surgeon Henry O'Hara purchased Cromwell House in 1892, and sold it in 1911. It later became the Alexandra Club (for women) and currently is the Melbourne fashion house of Louis Vuitton.

Returning to Abraham Lincoln's quote, with which I commenced this narrative, it is difficult in retrospect to separate the shadow of the man and the real thing, for there were controversies attached to both his character and his reputation. A medical historian, Dr. C. Craig, has described Beaney as 'egregious', i.e. distinguished in a bad sense (Webster) or outrageous (Oxford). Murray Morton, a surgeon nearer to his times, considered that he had many of the characteristics of a charlatan.

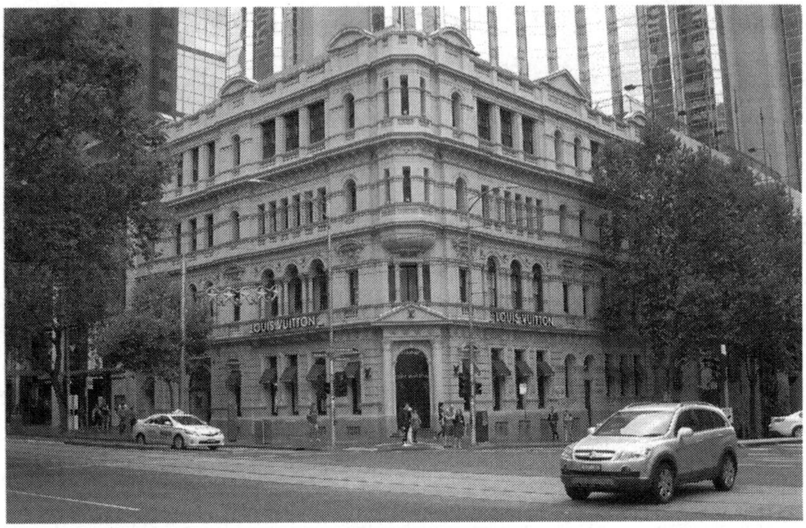

Figure 14: Louise Vuitton department store, Melbourne.

I do not regard him as totally unscrupulous but rather as an opportunist. Certainly he was an egotist but he was probably more often enterprising than dishonest in his professional life. An image Beaney would have liked is one that was conveyed in an acknowledgment (in a student publication) from one of his actual contemporaries: 'JGB is tough sir, devilish tough'.

The answer as to how such an undoubtedly ostentatious and indulgent man like James Beaney was tolerated in society and was successful is that much of society, at that time of sudden riches for so many, was equally so.

There are many inconsistencies both in this man and in his contemporary society. Beaney was, for example, diligent in practising an operation on cadavers prior to performing the stone removal but carelessly amputated a leg at the wrong level (through diseased bone) at the first operation performed on that same fateful December 2nd 1875. There is also a report of his failing to visit, for over 18 hours, a Mr. Joske, a well-connected businessman, who was admitted to hospital with a severe head injury, despite repeated requests from the junior medical staff during that period. The man died and the event was written up in *The Age.* Beaney blamed a junior staff member, Dr. F Lawson, who felt compelled to write to the newspaper to defend himself in a clarification of his own role in the patient's management.

Some uncertainty must remain also with regard to the role Beaney did or did not play in the death of the barmaid Mary Lewis. It is likely that she was pregnant as her uterus was enlarged to around '20 weeks'. It is not unusual that she would have consulted James Beaney about the pregnancy; as for some years after he returned to Melbourne he had continued to practice obstetrics, which had been a significant part of the practice he took over from Dr. Maund. We shall never know whether Mary Lewis requested Beaney to abort the pregnancy or assist in antenatal care, but I am inclined to favour the former reason.

It was a time of inconsistencies. Melbournians established fine roads and parks but accepted industrial slums and a grossly polluted Yarra River. Each had a saving grace, however. With Beaney it was his overt generosity and lasting endowments, although he left nothing in his will for his sister nor for his older brother George, who remained in Canterbury in poor circumstances, working as a labourer, as their father had. With our city forebears the saving grace was the outstanding architecture they have bequeathed to us, funded from the rivers of gold, which flowed south to Melbourne from Ballarat and Bendigo.

Returning to the operation of lithotomy it had since its inception, as indicated earlier, carried a significant risk to life. The originator of the lateral approach, Jacques Beaulieu, a medically unqualified Frenchman, reported at the end of the 17th century that, of 60 patients he had operated upon for stone, 25 had died and 13 were cured, but the remaining patients were incontinent and still in hospital. Subsequent to the publication of these results, and the ensuing criticism, he became despondent and adopted the habit of a monk. Then some years later, having more thoroughly studied anatomy and modified the operation by using a grooved staff, he reported on a further 38 patients, all of whom survived. However it was probably his early results that led to the well-known nursery rhyme:

> Frère Jacques, Frère Jacques,
> Dormez vous? Dormez vous?
> Sonnez les matines, Sonnez les matines,
> Ding dong ding, Ding dong ding.

William Cheselden, who was quoted by Purves during the inquest, was regarded as the foremost lithotomist of his time in any country, having further modified the operation of perineal lithotomy early in the 18th century. He reported operating on 212 patients, with a mortality rate of approximately 10%.

In contrast lithotomy from above, i.e. the suprapubic operation, which was suggested as an alternative procedure for Dr. Beaney to adopt, had been shown in the mid-19th century by Dr. Murray Humphrey, a Cambridge surgeon, to be associated with a 30% mortality rate. Hence it was reasonable for Beaney, particularly knowing of Berth's contracted bladder, to avoid that approach.

Sir John Erichsen, was another eminent surgeon, whose writings were quoted by Purves. Erichsen's best-known textbook was *Science and Art of Surgery,* which went through many editions. His reputation was worldwide and he was considered to be among the developers of "modern" surgery. However he was quoted as saying in 1873 that 'The abdomen, the chest and the brain will be forever shut from the wise and humane surgeon.' This fits well with the first of Arthur C Clarke's Three Laws:

> When a distinguished but elderly scientist states that something is possible, he is almost certainly right. When he states that something is impossible, he is very probably wrong.'

There was a remarkable and unexplained fall in the incidence of primary bladder stone in Western countries from the 19th to the 20th centuries, almost disappearing in children, but remaining prominent in various Asian societies. The earliest bladder stone, found in the grave of an Egyptian boy just sixteen years of age, was thought to date from 4,800BC. It was presented to the Royal College of Surgeons Hunterian Museum in London in 1901 and was 2.6 inches (6.5cm) in diameter.

Incidentally, there was a report in *The Lancet,* in August 1867, of the removal of a much larger stone than the one Dr. Beaney prized. Dr. John Burns of Glasgow operated upon a thirty-five-year-old man by the lateral approach and, using much traction, removed the stone. Despite injuring the rectum he reported that the patient made a full recovery without any complications (probably untrue). The stone weighed 6 3/4 ounces and measured 9 by 7 1/2 inches!

I wonder if James Beaney had read that report.

Bibliography

Background information was obtained from many sources. In addition to the publications referred to in the text, sources included:

Bartlett G.R. *Political Organization and Society in Victoria. 1864-188.* (Canberra: Australian National University, 1964).

Bate W.A. *The History of Brighton.* (Melbourne: Melbourne University Press. 1962).

Blaney G. *The Rush that never ended: a History of Australian Mining.* (Melbourne: Melbourne University Press, 1963).

Burchett W. *East Melbourne 1837-1977 People, Places, Problems.* (Hawthorn, Victoria: Craftsman Press. 1978).

Cannon M. *Melbourne after the Gold Rush.* (Main Ridge, Vic: Loch Haven Books, 1993).

Cannon M. *The Land Boomers.* (Melbourne: Melbourne University Press, 1966).

Davidson G. *The Rise and Fall of Marvellous Melbourne.* (Melbourne: Melbourne University Press, 1978).

Dunstan K. *The Paddock that Grew.* (London: Cassell & Co, 1962).

Ellis H.A. *A History of Bladder Stone.* (London: Blackwell Scientific Publications Ltd, 1969).

Grant J. and Serle G. *The Melbourne Scene 1803 to 1956.* (Melbourne: Melbourne University Press, 1957).

Goad P. *Melbourne Architecture.* (Borowa, NSW: The Watermark Press, 1999).

Gregory A. *The Ever Open Door – A History of the Royal Melbourne Hospital.* (Melbourne: Hyland House Publishing, 1998).

Hall A R. *The Stock Exchange of Melbourne and the Victorian Economy 1852 to 1900.* (Canberra: ANU Press, 1968).

Harvey A. *The Melbourne Book.* (Richmond, Vic: Hutchinson of Australia, 1982).

Lemon A. *The Northcote Side of the River.* (Melbourne: Hargreen Publishing, 1983).

Meudell G. *The Pleasant Career of a Spendthrift.* (London: George Rutledge & Sons, 1929).

Mitchell A.M. *The Hospital south of the Yarra: a History of Alfred Hospital.* (Melbourne: Melbourne University Press, 1977).

Newnham W.H. *Melbourne: Biography of a City.* (Melbourne: F W Cheshire, 1958).

O'Sullivan J.S. *A Most Unique Ruffian: The Trial of FB Deeming. Melbourne 1892.* (Melbourne: F W Cheshire, 1968).

Pensabene T.S. *The Rise of the Medical Practicioner in Victoria.* (Canberra: ANU Press, 1980).

Priestly S. *South Melbourne: A History.* (Melbourne: Melbourne University Press, 1995).

Rimmer W.G. *Portrait of a Hospital. The Royal Hobart Hospital.* (Hobart: Hobart RHH, 1981).

Russell K.F. *The Melbourne Medical School 1862 to 1962.* (Melbourne: Melbourne University Press, 1977).

Scott E. *Historical Memoir of the Melbourne Club.* (Melbourne: Speciality Press, 1936).

Scott E. *A History of the University of Melbourne.* (Melbourne: Melbourne University Press in association with Oxford University Press,1936).

Serle A.G. *The Golden Age: A History of the Colony of Victoria. 1851-1861.* (Melbourne: Melbourne University Press, 1963).

Shaw M.T. *Builders of Melbourne. The Cockrams and their Contemporaries 1853-1972.* (Melbourne: Cypress Books, 1972).

Tipping M. *Melbourne on the Yarra.* (Melbourne: Lansdowne Publishing, 1978).

Twopeny R.E.N. *Town Life in Australia 1883.* (London: Penguin, 1973).

Weber A.F. *The Growth of Cities in the Nineteenth Century.* (New York: Macmillan Company, 1899).

Westgarth W. *Half a Century of Australian Progress: a Personal Retrospect.* (London: Sampson Low & Son, 1889).

Other sources included medical journals, particularly *The Lancet* and the *Australian Medical Journal* (now the *Medical Journal of Australia*) and the first seven volumes of the *Australian Dictionary of Biography.*

Back Cover Material

The setting is the city of Melbourne in the latter half of the 19th century, when it grew rapidly, due to the extensive amount of gold flowing from mid-Victoria. It concerns Dr James Beaney, a very colourful and controversial surgeon, who amassed a fortune from his practice, and displayed it in the jewellery he wore. He was, however, a generous benefactor to the Melbourne University and hospitals in Melbourne, as well as to his birthplace, the city of Canterbury in Kent. Beaney, not for the first time, after his re-appointment to the Melbourne Hospital was implicated in a court case following the death of a patient he had operated on for a large bladder stone. The inquest is outlined in considerable detail and the skill displayed by James Purves, the brilliant young barrister who defended him, will be evident to the reader.

"One of the most interesting and enjoyable books I have read for some time. Beaney was a colourful character in a booming time in Melbourne, and this has been brought splendidly to life by Brian Collopy."

–Professor Sir Peter Morris, AC, FRS, FRCS, Nuffield Professor of Surgery Emeritus, University of Oxford

Made in United States
Orlando, FL
04 November 2026

90202363R00186